The Chronic Prostatitis 360 Protocol

The Scientifically Proven Natural Treatment Protocol for Chronic Prostatitis

By
Philip Potasiak

Protocol 360 Media

Dedication

This book is dedicated to the men who struggle daily with the pain of chronic prostatitis.

Author and Publisher Note

Every effort has been made to ensure that the information contained in this book is complete and accurate. However, neither the publisher nor the author is engaged in rendering professional advice or services to the individual reader. The ideas, procedures, and suggestions contained in this book are not intended as a substitute for consulting with your physician or a qualified professional. All matters regarding your health require medical supervision. Neither the author nor the publisher shall be liable or responsible for any loss or damage allegedly arising from any information or suggestions in this book.

Copyright © 2025 Philip Potasiak
All Rights Reserved

Prostatitis 360 ® is a Service Mark of Philip Potasiak registered in the United States Trademark Office.

Without limiting the rights under the copyright reserved above, no part of this publication may be reproduced, stored in, or introduced into a retrieval system or transmitted in any form or any other means (electronic, mechanical, photocopy, recording, or otherwise) without the prior written permission of both the copyright owner and the above publisher of this book.

Printed in the United States

ISBN 979-8-9927375-0-9

Cover Design by Ruth H.

First Edition

Acknowledgments

This book is the result of five years of research. It is based on hundreds of scientific studies done by medical researchers around the world during the past 50 years. I relied solely on scientific studies that met the standards of rigorous scientific research and were published in peer-reviewed journals, including the most respected medical journals in North America, Europe, and Asia. Most of the researchers responsible for these scientific studies have dedicated their professional lives to researching conventional medical treatments and natural alternative treatments for chronic prostatitis, prostatitis Lower Urinary Tract Syndrome (LUTS), and pelvic floor dysfunction.

I want to acknowledge the important contributions of several researchers who had the greatest impact on the development of the Chronic Prostatitis 360® Protocol. They include Dr. J. Curtis Nickel at Queen's University in Canada and Dr Daniel Shoskes at the Cleveland Clinic in the US, two of the most prominent and prolific researchers of chronic prostatitis in the world. Some of the other important researchers include Dr Kirshner-Hermanns in Germany, Dr. Gallo in Italy, and Dr Qin in China, among many others. The book cites a total of over 200 scientific studies by over 100 medical researchers. They are, in some ways, the informal "co-authors" of this book. Without their important scientific research, this book, the Chronic Prostatitis 360 Protocol, and the cure for my chronic prostatitis symptoms would not have been possible.

Table of Contents

Acknowledgments iv

Important Disclaimer - Please Read vi

Part I Starting of the Process 1

Introduction 2

CHAPTER 1 Understanding Chronic Prostatitis 23

CHAPTER 2 Chronic Prostatitis and the American Healthcare System 62

CHAPTER 3 Conventional Medical Treatment for Chronic Prostatitis 84

PART II The Core Protocol 100

CHAPTER 4 The Chronic Prostatitis 360 Protocol Diet 101

Chapter 5 Supplements for Chronic Prostatitis 127

CHAPTER 6 Chronic Prostatitis Lifestyle Changes 166

Part III Advanced Chronic Prostatitis Treatment 183

CHAPTER 7 Chronic Pain Management 184

CHAPTER 8 Chronic Prostatitis Urination Symptoms 200

CHAPTER 9 Erectile Dysfunction and Chronic Prostatitis 219

CHAPTER 10 Chronic Prostatitis and Depression 249

Part IV Going Forward 282

CHAPTER 11 The Future of the Chronic Prostatitis 360 Protocol 283

Appendix I Chronic Pelvic Floor Dysfunction 294

APPENDIX II Foods and Drinks that irritate the bladder 309

REFERENCES 312

About the Author 354

Index 355

Important Disclaimer - Please Read

The materials presented in *The Chronic Prostatitis 360® Protocol: The Scientifically Proven Natural Chronic Prostatitis Treatment Protocol* are designed to provide information about largely natural treatments for chronic prostatitis. The information is for educational purposes only and is not intended to diagnose or treat any illness, disease, or medical condition. Before acting on the information presented in this book, the reader agrees that it is their sole responsibility to consult a licensed medical professional to determine whether such information is suitable for them. They should review any special health concerns, risk factors, or medical conditions—especially if they are currently taking prescription medication or undergoing treatment for a medical condition—to determine whether the foods, phytochemicals, supplements, nutrients, herbs, products, physical exercises, or other actions recommended or presented in this book are appropriate, in the correct amounts, or contraindicated based on the medications they are taking or any conditions related to them, as determined by their doctor or relevant medical authorities.

Part I

Starting of the Process

Introduction

I wrote this book for men struggling with chronic prostatitis, those who love them, and the urologists and medical professionals who want to help them. If you're a man struggling with chronic prostatitis, I am one of you. I lived with the daily pain of severe chronic prostatitis for years. I understand the devastating physical, emotional, and psychological consequences of this condition. What started out as my desperate search to stop my daily severe pain and urination problems grew and evolved into a complete science-based treatment protocol, a book, and a mission to help men like you suffering from chronic prostatitis. My message to you is simple. A dramatic improvement in your symptoms and, in many cases, a cure is possible even if you have serious chronic prostatitis symptoms, as I did. There are scientifically proven treatments that work, and they have been proven to work for millions of men in Europe and Asia during the past two decades.

Conventional Medical Treatments in the US don't Work

The stark reality of conventional medical treatment for chronic prostatitis in the US is that it doesn't work. Medical research, patient outcomes, and the clinical experience of urologists confirm this. I developed the Chronic Prostatitis 360® Protocol and wrote this book after trying a wide range of traditional medical treatments and finding that none of them worked. In fact, some traditional medical treatments, such as the use of antibiotics for the treatment of chronic prostatitis, can do more harm than good. Although the medical establishment in the US has widely discredited antibiotics as a treatment for chronic prostatitis, many urologists continue to use them. During the first two years that I struggled with chronic

Introduction

prostatitis, I saw six urologists. I tried at least one of the drugs in all five classes of drugs and the two primary medical procedures used to treat chronic prostatitis. They were all completely ineffective. There are, however, some conventional medical treatments that are somewhat effective. Most urologists are not familiar with these treatments and, therefore, don't use them. They are not as effective as the supplements in the Chronic Prostatitis 360 Protocol, but they do deserve consideration, and they are part of the protocol options discussed in the book.

It's important to recognize, however, that while conventional medicine does not play, for the most part, a direct role in treating chronic prostatitis, it does play a very important role in the overall management of the condition. We need primary care doctors, urologists, and other specialists to do the initial and ongoing testing to confirm the diagnosis and rule out other causes or major contributing factors. We also need traditional medicine to treat underlying conditions that may be contributing factors to our chronic prostatitis. Conventional medical care is also important in treating depression and sexual problems, which are common side effects of chronic prostatitis.

US Compared to Europe

The situation in Europe, on the other hand, is very different. One of the three major components of the Prostatitis 360 Protocol, scientifically proven supplements, has been gradually incorporated into mainstream medical and urology practice in Europe during the past 25 years. Many urologists in Europe use phytotherapy (flower pollen, saw palmetto, nettle root, pumpkin seed oil) just as readily as prescription drugs or any other treatment approach. In Germany, to cite just one example, 50% of urologists use the supplement saw palmetto as a first-line treatment, they turn to for chronic prostatitis, and 90% use it as the first treatment for benign prostate enlargement, which is commonly abbreviated as BPH.

Benign prostatic hyperplasia, or BPH, is the medical term for benign prostate enlargement. They use a special type of saw palmetto berry extract called LESRSr saw palmetto extract. This special version of saw palmetto is inexpensive and readily available over the counter in the US without a prescription. The other supplements widely used in Europe include flower pollen, nettle root extract, and pumpkin seed oil. All of these are a category of supplements called phytotherapies. They are among the key treatments for chronic prostatitis in the Chronic Prostatitis 360 Protocol. In short, scientifically proven supplements and, in some cases, diet and lifestyle changes have been integrated into the mainstream of chronic prostatitis treatment by urologists and the medical establishment in Europe.

In Europe, flower pollen, saw palmetto, nettle root and pumpkin seed oil are recognized by medical establishment as drugs and manufactured by pharmaceutical companies in Sweden, Germany, France, Spain, and Italy.

The consequences for men struggling with chronic prostatitis in the US during the past 25 years have been devastating. Millions of men who could have been helped have continued to live with debilitating daily pain, urination problems, and, in many cases, severe erectile dysfunction or ED and depression. Why this stark difference between the U.S. and Europe?

1. In Europe, the major phytotherapies that are used to treat chronic prostatitis are treated and regulated as drugs. They are manufactured and marketed by pharmaceutical companies, including, for example, the leading makers of

Introduction

saw palmetto in France, Italy, and Germany. There is, therefore, greater trust in these three treatments by doctors, patients, and the medical establishment. These phytotherapies are considered supplements in the US; they are largely unregulated and made by supplement companies. There is less trust in supplements in the US. Doctors in the U.S., including urologists, often argue that supplements are ineffective or even dangerous. There is a general bias against supplements in the medical establishment in the US. There are a few exceptions; for example, hospitals in the US routinely give patients the supplement melatonin as a sleep aid, and doctors routinely recommend prenatal supplements to pregnant women. When the medical establishment accepts supplements, they are widely used in the US. For men with chronic prostatitis in the US, supplement use requires greater attention to selecting independently tested and proven products by reputable brands. However, it is possible to find safe and effective supplement brands. I discuss these brands in the book. The concerns about supplement safety and quality are not an obstacle to successfully and safely using them to treat chronic prostatitis in the US.

2. Scientifically proven supplements for the treatment of chronic prostatitis are recognized at the European and EU levels and the individual country level by regulatory agencies that are the European equivalents of the FDA and AUA in the US. Urologists, urology treatment centers, health insurance providers, and the public healthcare systems common in Europe can all make chronic prostatitis treatment decisions by using scientifically proven supplements approved by local and European health

authorities. In the US, the FDA and related federal health agencies are legally prohibited from regulating supplements by laws passed in Congress in the early 1990's. FDA approval or the lack of it does not explain alone why supplements are not widely used to treat chronic prostatitis in the US. Hospitals use the melatonin supplement as a sleep aid, and doctors routinely prescribe prenatal supplements without FDA approval. However, the official regulatory recognition of supplements in Europe as treatments for chronic prostatitis has made the widespread adoption of these supplements during the past 25 years much easier. This is an important difference between the US and Europe.

3. We have a for-profit healthcare system in the US. Doctors in the US cannot make a living (generate revenue and make a profit) recommending or "prescribing" supplements, diet, and lifestyle changes. They must write prescriptions for drugs and perform medical procedures. A urologist in the US has no economic incentive to read research on supplements, diet, and lifestyle change as treatments for chronic prostatitis. There has been, in fact, a great deal of research on the effectiveness of supplements in treating chronic prostatitis published in the major urology journals in the US. The primary audience for these journals is urologists, but again, they have no incentive to read this research, and judging by how few of them know about supplements for chronic prostatitis, they don't read the research. In our for-profit healthcare system, urologists often make treatment decisions, in the case of chronic prostatitis, based on what is profitable rather than what is proven to be effective when treating chronic prostatitis.

Introduction

4. Most European countries, in contrast, have not-for-profit healthcare systems, and therefore, doctors have much greater freedom in treating patients with what works, including supplements, rather than focusing on what generates revenue and profit. Doctors and their supervisors, in fact, have powerful incentives to read research in the major urology journals about scientifically proven supplements for the treatment of chronic prostatitis. In not-for-profit healthcare systems, doctors and healthcare systems have a greater focus on successful patient outcomes rather than revenue and profit. They do have to focus on controlling costs (just as in the US), but here, supplements, diet, and lifestyle changes are much less expensive than prescription drugs and medical procedures.

5. The supplement markets in the US and Europe are also very different. In the US, there are hundreds of supplements that claim to treat or help with "prostate" and "urination" health issues. But they almost invariably don't have a high enough dose of the proven phytotherapies for chronic prostatitis and, in many cases, only have one or two of them, usually quercetin and saw palmetto. Therefore, to the extent men turn to supplements, the supplements they find available in the US are almost invariably ineffective in treating chronic prostatitis. In Europe, the small number of supplements for chronic prostatitis include the main phytotherapies in the proper dose to be effective. I discuss how to use phytotherapy to treat chronic prostatitis in Chapter 5 successfully.

6. Most doctors in the US can't help; most supplements available in the US are ineffective, and when men turn to the Internet for information about the treatment of chronic prostatitis, they find very little or no information about treatments that are effective on the most popular health information websites. All the information about proven treatments is there. There is, in fact, a vast collection of research on scientifically proven treatments for chronic prostatitis done during the past 40 years. The key is to know how to search for it using the right search terms. I discuss these search techniques in chapters 2 and 3.

It's important to note that while most European countries are far ahead of the US in the adoption of the leading phytotherapy for the treatment of chronic prostatitis, there is a great deal of variation from country to country in Europe and among individual practicing urologists in those countries. While it does happen, it is not yet common for urologists who use supplements to treat chronic prostatitis and also to integrate diet and lifestyle changes to create a complete treatment program comparable to the Chronic Prostatitis 360 Protocol. Supplements are the single most important treatment for chronic prostatitis. They can and have provided significant improvement to many men in Europe. In some cases, they can provide dramatic improvement, especially if their symptoms are mild. However, for most men with more severe symptoms, supplements alone can't provide a dramatic improvement. In all cases, most men will need the complete Prostatitis 360 Protocol to achieve a cure or come close to a cure. In other words, supplements are a great start, but most urologists in most European countries do not offer a complete chronic prostatitis treatment protocol that most

Introduction

men need. That's why I plan to write a European edition of this book that will be adapted to the circumstances and needs of men with chronic prostatitis in Europe.

Finally, it's important to note that the differences between the US and Europe in the treatment of chronic prostatitis are ultimately the result of historical, cultural, and systemic differences that explain many of the specific individual differences discussed above and many more. Ultimately, to truly understand why Europe has adopted successful treatments for chronic prostatitis during the past 25 years that have not been adopted in the US, we would have to do a detailed analysis of the historical, cultural, and systemic differences between Europe and the US. We would have to look at things such as the nature of medical education in the US and Europe, the long history of the use of herbs and phytotherapy to treat medical conditions in Europe, the power and influence of the pharmaceutical and supplement industries in the US and many more topics that are beyond the scope of this book.

Are Alternative Treatments Credible?

Virtually every aspect of the dominant conventional health care system in the US either almost entirely ignores, doesn't know about, or disparages alternative treatments for chronic prostatitis. Almost everywhere man with chronic prostatitis turn to for help or information about treating their condition, the traditional health care system, almost all supplements available in the US, almost all common and popular sources of health information online, and online chronic prostatitis forums and chat groups all largely ignore proven alternative treatments for chronic prostatitis. I believe that this creates a credibility challenge for alternative treatments for chronic prostatitis for anyone who claims that there are effective treatments or a cure for chronic prostatitis. It's hard to believe. How is this possible? Is it possible that there are proven treatments that work, but they're not available in the US, and no one seems to know about them? Is it possible that they've been available for 25 years? Is it possible they have been successfully used for over 25 years in Europe, and no one seems to know about them here in the US? Is it possible that most urologists in the US, the experts in treating chronic prostatitis, don't offer or don't know about these treatments? I think these are all very logical reactions to the situation we face in the treatment of chronic prostatitis in the US. That's why I focused a great deal in the section above on the differences between the US and Europe and how those differences help to explain their very different approach to alternative treatments. That's why I devote a great deal of this book to documenting and discussing in detail the medical research that provides scientific evidence for the effectiveness of these alternative treatments.

Finally, it's important to acknowledge that there are urologists in the US and Canada who are widely recognized around the world as experts in treating chronic prostatitis who have extensively studied alternative treatments and who advocate the use of supplements such as quercetin, saw palmetto, pollen, and others. However, they have had little impact on most practicing urologists, patients, or the wider urology establishment in the US. Most of them are researchers in academic settings. Two prominent examples are Dr. J. Curtis Nichols at the University of Toronto and Dr. Daniel Shoskoes at the Cleveland Clinic. In terms of impacting the urology establishment and chronic prostatitis treatment, they've had a greater impact in Europe.

Scientific Research

This book is the result of the research done by hundreds of medical researchers from around the world. What I call the Chronic

Introduction

Prostatitis 360 Protocol draws on the work of hundreds of researchers from around the world during the past 50 years. As the author of this book, I didn't invent, create, or develop any new treatment. What I did do was assemble or bring together in one place the most effective, rigorous, proven scientific research on how to treat chronic prostatitis into a complete treatment plan, program, and step-by-step guide, what medical professionals call a protocol. In the process of finding a cure for my chronic prostatitis, I read hundreds of research reports and scientific studies. This book has over 200 references to specific scientific studies. Every treatment component in the protocol and analysis of the nature of the treatment of chronic prostatitis is backed up, documented, referenced, and footnoted with rigorous scientific research. All the major treatments in the protocol, including supplements, diet, and lifestyle changes, are documented with scientific proof that they are effective in treating the symptoms of chronic prostatitis. The protocol is based on hundreds of RCT studies involving thousands of men with chronic prostatitis in the US and around the world. Randomly Controlled Trials, or RCTs, are the standard used by medical researchers and medical professionals to define a rigorous scientific study. The highest standard or "gold standard" for a scientific study is a randomized, placebo-controlled double crossover stage 3 and 4 trials. One or two RCT studies are not enough to meet the definition of rigorous scientific research. There must be multiple studies with comparable results. Once there are multiple studies, medical researchers do a meta-analysis, which is an analysis and review of several RCT studies. Most of the studies I relied on to develop the protocol involved multiple studies and meta-analyses. In fact, if a particular treatment only had one or two studies, I left it out unless the results were particularly compelling, in which case, I say that early research is promising, but more studies are needed. I'm not a medical professional, I'm not a medical researcher, and I haven't done original scientific research. I didn't have to. All the RCT studies and related information I used to write this book and to formulate the Chronic Prostatitis 360 Protocol were readily available on the Internet for free. My contribution to the protocol and the book was to assemble a complete, coherent protocol based on these studies and to add my insights and perspective as a man who lived with severe chronic prostatitis for years.

My Role as the Author

The fact that I am not a medical professional or medical researcher was, in fact, an advantage in developing the protocol and writing the book. Healthcare in the US is fragmented in the sense that conventional medicine rarely works with so-called alternative or complementary alternative medicine or CAM. These are largely two separate camps that don't interact with each other and, in many ways, regard each other with suspicion and distrust. It is also the nature of medical research in the US and around the world that medical researchers are highly focused on narrow specialists. And in fact, to be successful that's what they must do. The result is that they don't step back and look at a more holistic view of a complex medical condition like chronic prostatitis.

In the process of finding a treatment for my symptoms, developing a treatment protocol, and writing this book, I had the advantage of not belonging to any camp in the US healthcare system or being narrowly focused on any particular field of medical research around the world. I could, and I did, go around the world and evaluate the research done on drugs and supplements developed in the US and Europe, traditional Chinese medicine, ayurvedic medicine in India, prostate massage widely practiced in Russia, Turkey, and other countries, acupuncture as it's practiced around the

Introduction

world, diet, exercise, lifestyle changes and many more. I could, and I did ask the question: Is there rigorous scientific research to prove that it works? How well does it work? How does it compare to other treatments? How many rigorous scientific studies have been done to prove its effectiveness? Not having any particular mindset, conventional healthcare, alternative treatments, Chinese medicine, etc., has actually been an important advantage in developing the Chronic Prostatitis 360 Protocol and writing this book.

Importance of Diet First

One of the significant personal insights I bring to the protocol and the book is the idea that diet is the first step in the process of treating chronic prostatitis. I believe that an anti-inflammatory diet lays the foundation that makes all the other treatments more effective, especially phytotherapy and prescription drugs. There is a great deal of common sense and logic to back up this belief. Chronic prostatitis is the chronic inflammation of the prostate, urethra, and, in some cases, the bladder. The treatments for chronic prostatitis, including supplements, drugs, diet, and lifestyle changes, among others, are in one way or another directly or indirectly designed to counter and reduce this inflammation in the body, including the prostate, urethra, and bladder. Highly inflammatory foods such as alcohol, caffeine, and hot/spicy foods are daily inflammation assaults on the body, including inflammation of the prostate. If you've had a lifetime of consuming highly inflammatory foods, it will take a minimum of 45 to 90 days for the damage caused by this long-term daily inflammation assault to begin to heal, and it may take up to six months for your body to fully recover. When I tried taking flower pollen and quercetin prior to starting an anti-inflammation diet, there was no benefit after 75 days. However, after implementing the diet, when I tried flower pollen again, I began to see some benefits after just 30 days and significant benefits after 60 days. After 90 days and beyond, I saw a dramatic improvement, and it proved to be one of the two most effective treatments for my chronic prostatitis. Your results will vary. You may find that flower pollen provides very little benefit, while quercetin and saw palmetto prove to be the most effective. I believe that there's a great deal of variation among men in their chronic prostatitis, and what provides a great deal of benefit for one man may provide little benefit for another and vice versa. Why? We don't know. Why do men go on for decades eating highly inflammatory foods without any obvious consequences and suddenly find at age 40, 50, or 60 that this diet is an important contributing factor to their chronic prostatitis? Again, we don't know. There is a great deal about chronic prostatitis that is baffling to patients, doctors, and medical researchers.

However, I believe that the role of diet as the foundation for chronic prostatitis treatment protocol is likely to be the one universal aspect of the protocol. Had I started with the major scientifically proven supplements for chronic prostatitis before implementing an anti-inflammatory diet, I may have falsely concluded that these supplements simply don't work in my case and given up. This would have had devastating consequences for my success with the protocol because four of the supplements proved to be the most important parts of the protocol in treating my chronic prostatitis. If not for these four supplements, I would have achieved approximately 30%, perhaps 40% improvement with the rest of the protocol, but I would never have achieved a complete cure. A 40% improvement in my severe daily pain and urination problems would have been a significant improvement in my symptoms, but of course, it's a far cry from a complete cure.

I believe there is an important lesson here for each man reading this book. What works for one man will not work the same way for

Introduction

another. You may find, for example, that diet provides a significant improvement but that supplements don't work until you implement an aerobic exercise program or one of the other lifestyle changes. The chronic Prostatitis 360 Protocol is a step-by-step process, but it's not a detailed blueprint that every man follows in exactly the same way with the same outcome. The protocol is a framework that you follow but adapt based on your own individual experience with each step in the process. The protocol is a process that involves some level of trial and error. You have to take the protocol and continue to experiment with what works for you in the order that it works for you. The protocol lays out a basic framework that starts with diet followed by supplements and lifestyle changes with treatment plans for pain, urination symptoms, erectile dysfunction, and psychological health as needed after implementing the program. If you follow the protocol in the order in the book and use a daily diary to monitor your symptoms, you can determine which components of the protocol are more or less effective and focus on what works for you. In my case, the diet changes reduced my symptoms by approximately 30%, followed by supplements, which reduced my symptoms by another 60%, and the other lifestyle changes, which provided the remaining 10% improvement. Your results will almost certainly be different. You may, for example, see a 20% benefit from diet, a 40% benefit from supplements, and a 40% benefit from some or all of the lifestyle changes. It took me 24 months to fully implement and see the full benefits of the protocol. It took longer because I was researching and building the protocol as I went. Most men should be able to complete the protocol in 6 to 12 months and see the full benefit in approximately 18 months. You may be able to accomplish the same thing in 6 months, or it may take 18 months in your case. To be successful, the protocol requires patience and the ability to adapt to a great deal of change.

The Challenge of Change

Change is very difficult. Most of us find that making even one relatively small change is difficult. The chronic Prostatitis 360 Protocol involves a great deal of change for most men. The diet and lifestyle changes of the protocol involve a dramatic change for most adult men in the US. If we take a typical middle-aged man in the US who eats a classic American diet, who has been sedentary for a decade or more, who has one or two drinks every night after work, drinks coffee all day at work, who is struggling with the stresses of work, health, and family and who has had a beer belly for a decade just making the first two diet changes (stopping alcohol and caffeine) in the protocol may represent a major challenge. Implementing all the changes in the protocol in 6, 12, or even 18 months may simply feel overwhelming and seem impossible. I believe the only thing that will motivate a man like this to make these major changes is if he has been struggling with the severe daily pain of chronic prostatitis for years and believes that the Chronic Prostatitis 360 Protocol has a credible chance of working. That's one of the reasons I devote a great deal of the book to discussing the rigorous scientific studies that provide evidence that each of the components of the protocol is scientifically proven to be effective. That's one of the reasons the book is documented with 199 references to the scientific studies that form the basis for the protocol.

In short, not only is there rigorous scientific research to prove the effectiveness of the protocol, but there are also 25 years of real-world experience involving millions of men in Europe who have successfully used the treatments in the protocol. There is no greater level of evidence of the effectiveness of any treatment for a medical

Introduction

condition. But of course, what really counts is what happens when you implement the Chronic Prostatitis 360 Protocol.

Chronic Prostatitis vs Chronic Pelvic Floor Pain

This book is primarily dedicated to treatments for chronic prostatitis. There is another condition that is often confused with chronic prostatitis, which is usually referred to as pelvic floor dysfunction (PFD) and is also known as chronic pelvic pain syndrome or CPPS. CPPS is more generic chronic pelvic floor pain, and PFD is more precise. Chronic prostatitis and chronic PFD are two different conditions. Chronic prostatitis is a condition of the prostate, urethra, and bladder that primarily impacts men over 50. The main symptoms are pain in the prostate and urethra, and less often, the bladder, along with urination problems and, in approximately 60% of men, erectile dysfunction. Chronic pelvic floor pain, on the other hand, is a condition of the pelvic floor and surrounding areas of the lower pelvis characterized primarily by chronic pain of the pelvic floor muscles. The causes and treatment of these two conditions are very different. There is some overlap in symptoms such as erectile dysfunction, but even in this case, there are important differences. Men with chronic pelvic floor dysfunction often have painful ejaculation and/or premature ejaculation. Whereas men with chronic prostatitis typically have erectile dysfunction alone.

Men with chronic pelvic floor dysfunction are usually under 40. Urologists often confuse the two conditions, which can make initial diagnosis difficult. In Chapter 1, I focus on the testing and diagnosis of chronic prostatitis, PFD, and related conditions with similar symptoms. If, in the course of reading Chapter 1, you determine that you have chronic pelvic floor pain, Appendix I provides an introduction and outline of the treatment of chronic pelvic floor dysfunction. There's little to no research data on the prevalence of chronic PFD. All we have are the estimates of some experts in the field who believe that approximately 50% of men have chronic prostatitis and the other 50% have PFD.

Start Here and Start Now

The place to start the process of implementing the chronic prostatitis 360 protocol is with several critical steps to measure, monitor, and keep track of your chronic prostatitis condition and your overall health. Take the time now before you start reading Chapter 1 to start a daily health diary and complete the CPSS Questionnaire. If you have erectile dysfunction (ED), use the IEDSS questionnaire. Urination problems are a normal part of chronic prostatitis, but if your urination symptoms are severe, there is another questionnaire. If, for example, you need to urinate more than 2 times during sleep every night. There is the IPSS to measure the severity of urination symptoms.

The daily health diary is a spreadsheet you create to track every aspect of your health and your symptoms daily. There is a model daily health diary, and I discuss how to create and use the diary in Chapter 1. Medical researchers use the CPSS to measure the severity of prostatitis and distinguish between chronic prostatitis and chronic pelvic floor pain. Chronic prostatitis medical researchers use the CPSS to report results and determine the level of success. There's a copy of the CPSS questionnaire in Chapter 1. You can also download a PDF of the questionnaire by searching "CPSS.pdf" online. The CPSS establishes a detailed baseline of the severity of your chronic prostatitis and allows you to monitor your progress as you implement new treatments in the protocol. The health diary allows you to keep track of the impact of new treatments or any other aspect of your health and how they impact your chronic prostatitis symptoms and progress.

Introduction

How to Implement the Chronic Prostatitis 360 Protocol

The core Chronic Prostatitis 360 Protocol has three parts: diet changes, phytotherapy/supplements, and lifestyle changes, presented in chapters 4, 5, and 6. I recommend following the protocol in this order. It's particularly important to start the protocol with diet before going on to supplements. If, however, you have reason to believe that starting with exercise, sexual habits, or changing how long you sit may be a good idea, do so. If, for example, you have made changes in the level of aerobic exercise or changes in your sexual or sitting habits that you believe started or made your symptoms worse, it may make sense in your case to start there while at the same time implementing the diet stage of the protocol. It is important to start with the diet changes in the protocol, but beyond that, you should begin to implement the supplement and lifestyle changes as soon as you can and as quickly as you can without necessarily following a strict order. In other words, you don't have to complete implementing the supplement stage before starting lifestyle changes. Sometimes, intentionally or unintentionally, I tended to follow more of a sequential approach. I would implement a new treatment for 60 days without making any other changes to measure the effectiveness of that treatment. This was in part because I didn't have the protocol to follow; I was implementing a new treatment as I learned about it. Ideally, you would take 90 days to implement the diet and 60 days each for the three supplements and the lifestyle changes to measure the impact of these individual treatments and to know which is more effective and which is less effective or not effective at all. The challenge with this approach is that if you make just the diet changes, the three core supplements, and implement an exercise program for 90 days, it adds up to 12 months. For men struggling with severe chronic prostatitis pain, taking 12 months for what you can do in 6 months is not going to be an attractive option. These are just five parts of the protocol, and they don't include several other supplements, two traditional medical treatments, and several other lifestyle changes. I think most men will understandably take more of an "all of the above" approach to implementing the protocol as quickly as they can possibly implement multiple changes.

The book is organized into four parts. The three chapters in Part 1 focus on diagnosing chronic prostatitis, managing the limitations of the American healthcare system, and understanding the role of conventional medical care in treating chronic prosthetics. Part II has the core protocol, which has three stages that correspond to chapters 4,5 and 6. The final four chapters in Part III are for men who have achieved significant improvement with the protocol but continue to have pain, urination, ED/sexual health, and psychological health issues and need additional treatment options to resolve these issues. The final chapter of the book looks at the future of the Prostatitis 360 Protocol.

Part I: Getting Started
1. Understand, test, and measure your chronic prostatitis (Chapter 1)
2. Managing the Limitations of the American Healthcare System (Chapter 2)
3. The role of conventional healthcare (Chapter 3)

Part II: The Core Treatment Protocol
4. Start the diet stage of the protocol first (Chapter 4)
5. Implement the supplement stage (Chapter 5)
6. Make lifestyle changes (Chapter 6)

Introduction

> Part III: The Advanced Protocol
> 7. Treating Persistent Pain
> 8. Treatment for Persistent Urination Problems
> 9. Erectile Dysfunction Protocol
> 10. Depression Treatment Plan
>
> Part IV: Going Forward
> 11. The Future of the Prostatitis 360 Protocol

The 90-Day Quick Start Program

1. Read Chapter 1 to confirm a chronic prostatitis diagnosis. Start a daily health diary and do the CPSS questionnaire described in Chapter 1.
2. Start the diet stage by removing all forms of alcohol, caffeine (coffee/decaf, tea, chocolate), and hot & spicy foods from your diet (Chapter 4). There is much more, but you can start there.
3. Take the five core phytotherapy: quercetin, saw palmetto, flower pollen, nettle root, and pumpkin seed oil. Make sure you take the right brands, dosages, and versions of these five products discussed in Chapter 5.

You may begin to see some mild improvement after 90 days, but in most cases, it will take 120 or more days to see any significant improvement. These three quick, simple, and very basic steps are only starting points. Read the sections on the three supplements above for information about the right dosage, brands, and, in the case of saw palmetto and flower pollen, the right version to take. Most saw palmetto brands in the US, for example, are not effective in treating chronic prostatitis. If you decide to implement the Quick

Start program, it's important to read the entire book. Each chapter on diet, supplements, and lifestyle has details and nuanced information that can make a difference in achieving success or complete success with the protocol. There is no shortcut to success with the Prostatitis 360 Protocol, but if you have been suffering from severe chronic prostatitis pain for years, I can appreciate an intense desire to take immediate action. My concern is that you will not see immediate results and give up before taking the time and making the effort to implement the complete protocol. The protocol is not a quick cure. For the vast majority of men with chronic prostatitis, there is no quick cure. It will take 6 to 18 months to implement and see the full benefits of the protocol fully.

CHAPTER 1
Understanding Chronic Prostatitis

There are four types of prostatitis: Type I, II, III, and IV. The most common is Chronic Prostatitis or Type III. Chronic Prostatitis, or CP, is combined by medical researchers into a broader category or umbrella term for various forms of lower pelvic pain called Chronic Pelvic Pain Syndrome or CPPS, which includes chronic pelvic floor dysfunction. This combination is abbreviated as CP/CPPS and stands for Chronic Prostatitis / Chronic Pelvic Pain Syndrome. Researchers in the US and around the world use this abbreviation when discussing research on chronic prostatitis. The term prostatitis is often used as shorthand by urologists, primary care providers, and patients for both Chronic Prostatitis and Chronic Pelvic Floor Dysfunction. However, it is important to understand that chronic pelvic floor pain is a pelvic floor muscle condition not related to the prostate. Chronic prostatitis, in turn, is a prostate condition that is not related to the pelvic floor muscle.

Chronic Prostatitis

Prostatitis is a medical term that means "inflammation of the prostate." There are two types of prostatitis: bacterial prostatitis, either acute or chronic, and chronic non-bacterial prostatitis, which is normally just called chronic prostatitis. The prostate is a walnut-sized gland that is just below the bladder. The urethra is a narrow tube that runs from the bladder to the tip of men's penis that carries urine and passes through the prostate. Inflammation of the prostate and urethra irritates and puts pressure on the urethra, causing pain and painful or burning urination. The pain can also radiate to other parts of the lower pelvic area nearby, such as the testicles. Pain and urination symptoms, such as frequent urination, are the most common defining symptoms of prostatitis. Chronic prostatitis is the result of chronic inflammation of the prostate, urethra, and, in some cases, the bladder, which causes long-term chronic pain and urination symptoms. Most men, 90% to 95%, who have prostatitis have chronic prostatitis. The underlying cause or causes of the chronic inflammation of chronic prostatitis are unknown or poorly understood at best. However, a wide range of treatments for the symptoms of chronic inflammation have been extensively researched and proven to be effective in treating the symptoms of chronic prostatitis. It's the treatment of these chronic inflammation symptoms that is the basis of the Chronic Prostatitis 360 ® Protocol and the successful treatment of chronic prostatitis.

Chronic Pelvic Floor Dysfunction

Chronic Pelvic Floor Dysfunction is a chronic muscle tension disorder that is also known in the scientific community and among medical researchers as Chronic Pelvic Pain Syndrome or CPPS. The

CHAPTER 1
Understanding Chronic Prostatitis

term CPPS usually refers to chronic pelvic floor dysfunction, but it is also, in some cases, used as a more generic term for chronic pelvic pain related to other conditions or of unknown origin. Chronic pelvic floor dysfunction is a chronic muscle tension disorder that causes painful chronic muscle spasms primarily in the perineum or the pelvic floor area between the testicles and anus. It usually also causes chronic muscle tension and spasms in the muscles involved in ejaculation and bowel movements, and therefore, painful ejaculation and bowel movements are also common features of this condition. Chronic pelvic floor pain and chronic prostatitis both have some similarities in symptoms, such as urination symptoms, but they are fundamentally different. The defining symptoms of the two conditions are very different: chronic pelvic floor pain occurs in the pelvic floor and is caused by muscle tension, and chronic prostatitis is chronic prostate and urethra pain caused by inflammation. Chronic muscle tension in the pelvic floor is often described as the feeling of a clenched fist in the pelvic floor area that is painful and can't be relaxed. Appendix I provides a basic outline of a chronic pelvic floor pain treatment protocol. The rest of the book is dedicated to chronic prostatitis. Some researchers who are also practicing urologists believe, based on their clinical experience (office visits they receive), that pelvic floor dysfunction is as common as chronic prostatitis. In other words, the number of cases of chronic pelvic floor dysfunction is about the same as the number of cases of chronic prostatitis. The best evidence we have to support this assumption is studies that show that 16% of men have chronic prostatitis and 12.5% to 16% of men have pelvic floor dysfunction. Until rigorous scientific research is conducted, this is the best information we have about the distribution between chronic pelvic floor pain and chronic prostatitis. In short, the assumption is that approximately 50% of men have chronic prostatitis, and the other 50% have pelvic floor dysfunction. I use this working assumption throughout the book. We will explore this issue in greater detail in Chapter 2 because it impacts the way urologists understand and treat chronic prostatitis and the way physical therapists approach pelvic floor dysfunction.

Prevalence of Prostatitis

In the US, prostatitis affects 9% to 16% of the male population, with 8% to 9% being the most commonly used percentage. However, there is reason to believe that underreporting is a problem. One study found that only 60% of men seeking help for their chronic prostatitis to their doctors. **(1)** A study of medical professionals such as dentists and male nurses16% reported having prostatitis. Given the problem of underreporting, I believe that 16% of the results are likely to be more accurate. Prostatitis accounts for 11% of all urology patients in the US. It is responsible for 2 million doctor visits per year in the US, with treatment for the condition costing $84 million annually, not including prescription drugs. In one study, approximately 14% of men with a medical claim for prostatitis missed work. **(2)** This gives us some sense of the impact of prostatitis on patient quality of life and the economic impact of the condition. But there is a great deal we don't know. There are no large-scale comprehensive studies of the prevalence, economic, and personal impact of prostatitis. In the studies that have been done in the US and around the world, there is a wide variation in the statistics on the prevalence of the condition and little in-depth information on its economic impact. Finally, in terms of the impact on quality of life, we can only speculate about how prostatitis, especially for men with long-term chronic prostatitis

CHAPTER 1
Understanding Chronic Prostatitis

with severe symptoms, impacts their family life, marriages, psychiatric health, careers, and rates of disability. Experts in the field have often compared long-term chronic prostatitis to the devastating quality of life impact comparable to advanced-stage heart disease.

Prevalence by Age

In terms of prevalence by age, there is a commonly held belief among urologists and many in the urology community that prostatitis is a young man's disease or men under 40. This has been the conventional wisdom in the urology community for decades. On the other hand, the detailed, comprehensive studies of prevalence by age all conclude that prostatitis, especially chronic prostatitis, which is 90% to 95% of all cases, is a condition that impacts more men over 50 than under 50. A study by Wallner and colleagues of 703 men surveyed in person with a detailed questionnaire reported that 71% were over 50. **(3)**

A large population study involving 1,832 men in Finland done by Mehik and colleagues found that men from 50 to 59 are 3.1 times more likely to have prostatitis than men 20 to 39, while for men 40 to 49, it was 1.7 times more likely than men 20 to 39. **(4)** A Study of 2,115 men in Olmsted County, MN, by Roberts and colleagues found that overall, more men over 50 had chronic prostatitis than men under 50. In the Study, the peak decade was 30 to 39, and for men under 50 and men over 50, there was a sharp rise that began at 55 and continued to increase dramatically at age 60. The levels of chronic prostatitis for men in the 60s, 70s, and beyond were much higher than any decade for men under 50. **(5)** A 1998 study done by Collins and colleagues that analyzed a survey of 58,955 doctor visits between 1990 and 1996 reported 700,000 men under 50 were diagnosed with prostatitis compared to 900,000 men over 50 who were diagnosed with prostatitis. This study concluded that prostatitis is more common among men over 50. Yet this study is widely cited study as evidence that prostatitis is more common among younger men because the study observes that "Prostatitis is the most common urological diagnosis in men <50 years of age and is the third most common diagnosis among those >50 years of age" this statement does not mean that prostatitis is more common among younger men than older men it simply means that urological problems are much more common among older men and that one of the few common urological problems for younger men is prostatitis. Therefore, prostatitis is the most diagnosed urological problem for younger men because it's the only common urological problem that younger men have, with rare exceptions. There have been dozens of scholarly articles published about prostatitis in leading medical journals around the world that make the statement that prostatitis is more common among younger men that cite the Collins study to validate the statement when, in fact, the Collins study clearly states the opposite: that prostatitis is, in fact, more common among older men. As a result, the conventional wisdom that prostatitis is a "young man's disease" has stubbornly persisted despite the fact that the best available, most rigorous, and large-scale studies done during the past 40 years have consistently shown that, in fact, prostatitis is more common among men over 50.

Long-held traditional beliefs and conventional wisdom are very difficult to overcome. Ku and colleagues did a comprehensive review of prostatitis and chronic prostatitis prevalence by age with a careful analysis of 11 different studies of prostatitis and chronic prostatitis. In the study, the authors say that "Prostatitis has traditionally been considered a young man's disease." They go on

CHAPTER 1
Understanding Chronic Prostatitis

to present data from these studies showing that in nine of the 11 studies, more men over 50 had prostatitis or chronic prostatitis than men under 50, and in the two remaining studies, the number of men with prostatitis over 50 was the same as the number of men under 50. Despite the fact that the authors could not find a single study to substantiate the traditional belief that prostatitis is a young man's disease, they remained unwilling to declare that the young man's disease belief was inaccurate or a myth. They were also unwilling to acknowledge that most of the research they analyzed, in fact, showed that prostatitis was more common among older men. **(6)** This is not an arcane scholarly or academic issue. It has had and continues to have profound real-world consequences for the way primary care doctors, urologists, patients, and the urology establishment fail to understand, diagnose, and treat prostatitis, which we will discuss in greater detail in Chapter 2.

The Four Types of Prostatitis

There are four types of prostatitis, as defined by the US National Institutes of Health (NIH), which were adopted in 1999. It has since been the global standard for defining prostatitis.

Type I Acute Bacterial Prostatitis
Type II Chronic Bacterial Prostatitis
Type III Chronic Non-Bacterial Prostatitis, which is simply called Chronic Prostatitis
        Type III a. Inflammatory Chronic Prostatitis
        Type III b. Non-Inflammatory Chronic Prostatitis
Type IV Asymptomatic Prostatitis

Type III: Chronic Prostatitis

Chronic Prostatitis is known as Type III and is further divided into IIIA, or Inflammatory Chronic Prostatitis, and IIIB, or Non-inflammatory Chronic Prostatitis. The abbreviation CP/CPPS for Chronic Prostatitis / Chronic Pelvic Pain Syndrome is also widely used to describe chronic prostatitis, especially by scientific and medical researchers studying prostatitis. In Type III A Inflammatory Prostatitis, there is evidence of inflammation but not bacterial infection, which is detected in standard testing. The vast majority of men with chronic prostatitis have Type IIIB or non-inflammatory prostatitis without any evidence of inflammation in standard testing. The Prostatitis 360 treatment protocol is primarily focused on Chronic Prostatitis because this is the form of prostatitis most men have and because traditional medical treatment has proven to be largely ineffective in treating the condition. However, it's important to note that most treatments for non-inflammatory chronic prostatitis work equally well in most cases on inflammatory chronic prostatitis. In other words, in terms of treatment, including the Prostatitis 360 Protocol, there is little or no practical difference between the two types of chronic prostatitis.

The other three types of prostatitis are relatively easy to detect and treat using traditional or conventional medical care provided by urologists. They are:

Type I: Acute Bacterial Prostatitis
This is one of the easiest subtypes of prostatitis for physicians to diagnose. Acute bacterial prostatitis is caused by a bacterial infection that often happens quickly, and it can happen at any age, but it primarily affects younger men under 50. It normally includes a severe urinary tract infection accompanied by painful

CHAPTER 1
Understanding Chronic Prostatitis

urination or blocked urine flow, fever, lower back or abdominal pain, and vomiting. Acute bacterial prostatitis requires prompt treatment and may require a brief hospital stay in which you'll receive antibiotics, fluids, and catheter if urine flow is completely blocked. This type of prostatitis can be deadly if left untreated

Type II: Bacterial Prostatitis / Chronic Bacterial Prostatitis

This form of prostatitis is almost always caused by bacteria that are detected in standard testing and treated with antibiotics, which typically work well. The main challenge with bacterial prostatitis is that for some men, it becomes a recurring and, in rare cases, frequently recurring condition throughout their lives.

Type IV: Asymptomatic Inflammatory Prostatitis

Men with asymptomatic (without symptoms) inflammatory prostatitis usually don't experience any symptoms despite evidence of inflammation. The prostate is inflamed in this type of prostatitis, and evidence of inflammation can be found in the urine, semen, or fluids from the prostate that your doctor will want to take tests of to diagnose you. The true extent of this form of prostatitis is unknown because most men don't have symptoms, and as a result, it often goes underdiagnosed. However, studies of the autopsies of older men have found that a high percentage of men have prostatitis by the time they die in their 70s, 80s, and beyond. This suggests that chronic prostatitis may be much more common than is reported in prevalence studies either because men don't seek help or they don't have symptoms. It is another baffling aspect of prostatitis for patients, doctors, and medical researchers that some men with inflammation of the prostate never develop any symptoms, while many other men with chronic prostatitis often struggle with severe symptoms for years. The same baffling phenomenon occurs with men who have an enlarged prostate or BPH and never have any symptoms or the symptoms are so minor, such as a weaker urine flow, that they simply attributed them to "getting older" since most men with BPH are over 50 and the condition is more common as men age.

These other types of prostatitis are not directly addressed in this book. I think that men with recurring bacterial prostatitis could benefit from some aspects of Prostatitis 360, such as the Prostatitis 360 Diet, if conventional medical treatment is unsuccessful in addressing the frequent recurrence of bacterial prostatitis. But it's important to make clear that this is not supported by any scientific research at this point. As I emphasized throughout this book, rigorous scientific research is a critical guiding principle of this book and the chronic Prostatitis 360 Protocol.

Altogether, prostatitis types I, II, and IV are only 5% to 10% of all prostatitis cases. The majority of men with prostatitis, 90% to 95%, have chronic prostatitis, type III-A or B, and most of them, in turn, have non-inflammatory type III B chronic prostatitis.

Symptoms of Chronic Prostatitis

One of the many challenges of chronic prostatitis is the fact that evaluating the symptoms and determining the diagnosis of the condition can be very difficult. This is further complicated by the fact that urologists and the urology community in the US have lumped together chronic prostatitis and chronic pelvic floor dysfunction. In the minds of many urologists, chronic pelvic floor dysfunction is a type of prostatitis despite the fact that chronic pelvic floor dysfunction is not related to the prostate and is, therefore, NOT

CHAPTER 1
Understanding Chronic Prostatitis

a type of prostate inflammation or prostatitis. Nevertheless, many urologists use the generic term prostatitis to describe both men with chronic pelvic floor dysfunction and men with bacterial prostatitis, acute or chronic. And since chronic pelvic floor dysfunction and bacterial prostatitis are common among men under 40, they believe that prostatitis is a young men's disease. One of the urologists I saw insisted that I couldn't have prostatitis because I was over 50. He told me that prostatitis only affects younger men. He focused on doing tests to determine if I had BPH because some of the symptoms are similar and because BPH is common among men over 50. When the tests he conducted ruled out BPH, he offered no alternative diagnosis or theory for my symptoms, but he insisted it couldn't be prostatitis.

These two conditions are, in fact, two different conditions with very different symptoms, causes, testing, and treatments.

1. Chronic Prostatitis is caused by inflammation of the prostate. The primary defining dominant symptoms are pain in the prostate, urethra, and tip of the penis. The other major symptom is painful urination and urination problems such as frequent urination and weak urine flow. The dominant defining symptom is pain: prostate and urethral pain and painful urination. The pain can radiate to other parts of the pelvic region, such as the testicles, but these other pain symptoms are typically secondary, less severe causes of pain. In addition to pain and urination problems, approximately 60% of men with chronic prostatitis have erectile dysfunction or ED. Most men with Chronic prostatitis are over 50.

2. Chronic Pelvic Floor Dysfunction is caused by chronic stress and muscle tension. The dominant defining symptom is severe pelvic floor muscle pain which is the muscles located in the perineum (the area between the anus and the testicles) caused by chronic pelvic floor muscle spasms and tension. The pain can radiate to other parts of the lower pelvic region, most commonly the testicles and anus. Painful ejaculation is common and is the primary sexual health issue. Pelvic floor dysfunction diagnosis can sometimes be confusing for some men with the condition because some of them have many of the symptoms of chronic prostatitis, such as pain at the tip of the penis. What is critical for these men to remember is that their dominant defining pain is chronic pelvic floor pain caused by chronic pelvic floor muscle tension, and therefore, it's not chronic prostatitis. Most men with chronic pelvic floor dysfunction are, to the best of our knowledge, under 40, but it can occur at any age. Unfortunately, there is no reliable research data on prevalence by age.

If these conditions are so different, why include chronic pelvic floor pain in a book about chronic prostatitis? There is so much confusion about the two conditions among many urologists and patients that I concluded I couldn't discuss treating chronic prostatitis and ignore chronic pelvic floor dysfunction. Treating either condition starts with having a clear understanding of whether you have chronic prostatitis or chronic pelvic floor dysfunction. This book is primarily dedicated to treating chronic prostatitis because it's more complex and difficult to treat, and the condition was the

CHAPTER 1
Understanding Chronic Prostatitis

original inspiration for this book. I do, however, include in Appendix I an overview of the treatments for chronic pelvic floor pain.

Chronic Prostatitis

Chronic pain is the most important symptom of chronic prostatitis. In severe chronic prostatitis, the pain is severe, occurs daily, and is more or less constant throughout the day. These pain symptoms include pain in the urethra, the tip of the penis, prostate, and pain or a burning sensation during urination. It can radiate to other parts of the lower pelvic regions, including the testicles and bladder, but those symptoms are secondary. Urination symptoms are the other major indicator of chronic prostatitis, including pain and burning during urination, a weak urine flow, frequent urination, and the sensation that you still need to urinate after urinating. More severe urination symptoms, such as the inability to completely empty a full bladder and urinating four or more times overnight and 15 or more times during the day, are less common in chronic prostatitis. Pain during urination is a common symptom of the condition. If you have severe chronic prostatitis, the pain persists after urination. In the case of milder chronic prostatitis or on less severe days/times of the day for men with severe chronic prostatitis, urination provides complete or significant relief from the pain after urination. One of the indicators of severe chronic prostatitis is that urination provides very little or no relief. Erectile dysfunction (ED) is the third major symptom of chronic prostatitis and affects 60% to 70% of men with chronic prostatitis. Painful ejaculation can occur in some cases but is more common for men with chronic pelvic floor dysfunction, and ejaculation issues are typically limited to mild discomfort. Finally, chronic prostatitis often leads to depression, including severe or clinical depression.

If you use a pain scale of 1 to 5, with 1 being no pain or urination issues and 5 being very severe, the pain of severe CP tends to range from 3 to 5 on most days, and you only have rare days where the pain is 1 or 2 with 5 being extreme pain and 1 being normal or near normal. In my case, prior to starting the protocol, my pain typically ranged from 3 to 5. I never had a 1 day and very rarely had a 2 day, experiencing a 2 day every 30 to 40 days. The final indicator of CP is that your primary voiding symptom is a reduced urine flow rate, especially on severe pain days. But even on severe pain days, tests will show that you more or less fully empty your bladder. If you have an enlarged prostate (BHP) as opposed to inflammation of the prostate (chronic prostatitis), you will typically experience a wider range of urination symptoms and greater severity, including urgency, frequency, and urine retention in the bladder after urinating or in other words not fully emptying your bladder during urination in bladder urination retention tests. In severe BPH cases, the prostate becomes so enlarged that it totally blocks urine flow, and men must have a catheter inserted in the urethra up to the bladder to release urine backed up in the bladder, a procedure called catheterization.

The Prostatitis 360 1 to 5 pain scale.

I started using this 1 to 5 pain scale when I first began to track my symptoms. I found it much easier than trying to decide whether my pain was a 6 or a 7 on a scale of 1 to 10. if you need to convert the one-to-five scale to a one-to-10 pain scale, just multiply by two.

1: There is no pain all day. There may be mild pain or discomfort, but only during urination and briefly afterward.

CHAPTER 1
Understanding Chronic Prostatitis

1a: This is a near-normal day. But you experience some mild pain during part of the day.

2: Mild pain and urination symptoms. Urination provides significant relief. for 15 to 45 minutes.

3: Fairly severe pain and urination. Urine flow is slow and frequent. Urination provides only short-term relief.

4: The pain is very severe and constant from the time you wake up to the time you go to bed. Urine flow is very slow, limited in volume, and frequent. Urination provides no meaningful relief.

5: Pain is extreme and constant. This pain is debilitating, making it very difficult to focus, concentrate, or think about anything but your pain. This is a pain as bad as you can imagine.

To summarize, the following are the defining characteristics of chronic Prostatitis:

A. You experience pain most of the day or all day. Your primary pain is in the urethra, prostate, and during urination. These symptoms have persisted for 3 or more months. If you have severe chronic prostatitis, the pain ranges from 3 to 5 during most days of the month. If you have mild chronic prostatitis, it's 1.5 or 2.

B. Your urination symptoms are typically limited to a lower urine flow rate, pain, and burning during urination and more frequent urination, primarily during more severe pain days, that is, days where the pain is 3 or greater.

C. You may experience some discomfort during ejaculation, but pain, especially severe pain, is less common. ED is the primary sexual health issue in 60% to 70% of men.

If you have the 3 symptoms above, there is a very strong likelihood that you have chronic prostatitis if medical testing rules out other conditions with similar symptoms. And that your symptoms are caused by chronic inflammation of the prostate rather than some other condition such as BPH, overactive bladder, IC/PBS, or Interstitial Cystitis/Painful Bladder Syndrome. If you also have ED, that is consistent with a diagnosis of chronic prostatitis as well. If you combine this with a battery of tests discussed below to rule out BPH and other possible causes of your symptoms, you have the best currently available confirmation of a chronic prostatitis diagnosis.

How to diagnose Chronic Prostatitis? The 4-Step Process

You have chronic prostatitis if:

1. The two primary or dominant symptoms: A. Pain Symptoms: Pain in the prostate, urethra, and tip of the penis and painful/burning during urination. B. Urination Symptoms: Frequent day and nighttime urination, waking up to urination 2 or more times, slow urine flow, and sensation of still needing to urinate after urinating. Most men with chronic prostatitis also have ED, and some men have secondary symptoms such as pain in the testicles, but the dominant defining symptoms are severe chronic pain and urination symptoms outlined above. Finally, the symptoms are chronic (daily), and they have lasted for 3 or more months.

CHAPTER 1
Understanding Chronic Prostatitis

2. Your primary symptoms are **not** the symptoms of pelvic floor dysfunction. In other words, you do not have the dominant definition of severe chronic pain of the pelvic floor muscles or common secondary symptoms such as painful bowel movements and pain during ejaculation.
3. You have had the tests to rule out the causes of the symptoms: STDs, UTI, urethritis, and bacterial prostatitis. These tests are routinely done by primary care doctors for men with the symptoms of prostatitis.
4. The 3 key tests to rule out BPH confirm that you **do not** have an enlarged prostate:
    a. A bladder urine retention test is done by your primary care physician to determine if you fully empty your bladder when urinating.
    b. A urine flow test is used to measure the strength of your urine flow.
    c. Prostate ultrasound to measure the size of the prostate. Your urologist does these last two tests. These tests are critical to rule out BPH, which is the most common condition for men over 50 with similar symptoms to chronic prostatitis.

Optional step 5. Tests for rare conditions that have similar symptoms to chronic prostatitis. This step is only necessary in rare cases and is optional for most men.

For most men, if you have the symptoms above and you can rule out BPH and pelvic floor dysfunction, there is a very strong likelihood that you have chronic prostatitis rather than bacterial prostatitis or pelvic floor dysfunction and that your symptoms are caused by chronic inflammation of the prostate rather than some other condition such as enlarged prostate or BPH, overactive bladder or OAB and Interstitial Cytosis / Painful Bladder Syndrome or IC/PBS.

The Battery of Tests for Prostatitis & Chronic Prostatitis

There is no single test or combination of tests for diagnosing chronic prostatitis. It is a diagnosis of exclusion. If you have the defining symptoms of chronic prostatitis and you've completed the tests to exclude other likely causes of those symptoms, you have the best currently available confirmation of a chronic prostatitis diagnosis.

There are three very rare conditions that mimic the symptoms of chronic prostatitis. Theoretically, the tests to rule out these three conditions are the fifth step in the process of diagnosing chronic prostatitis, but in practice, because these conditions are so rare, most men can safely assume that the four steps discussed above are what they need for a diagnosis of chronic prostatitis. These three conditions and the tests to rule them out are discussed at the end of this section on testing. The following is the 5-step battery of tests for chronic prostatitis:

Step One: Initial Medical Testing & Preliminary Diagnosis

The symptoms of prostatitis, starting with pain, urination problems, and ED (in many cases), require a battery of tests that need to be conducted by your primary care doctor and urologist. Your primary care doctor should have conducted the following routine tests to rule out the most common causes of the pain and urination symptoms:

CHAPTER 1
Understanding Chronic Prostatitis

A. STD test to rule out a sexually transmitted disease.

B. Urine test to rule out UTI and urethritis or bacterial infections of the urethra.

C. Urine tests to rule out infections of the prostate or bacterial prostatitis (acute or chronic)

D. Bladder urine retention test to determine if BPH is a possible cause. This is the first of 3 tests to rule out BPH. A Urologist does the other two.

E. PSA blood test to rule out prostate cancer.

If the basic tests above come back negative, you should be referred to a urologist for advanced testing. The three tests in step two below should be completed during your initial visit with the urologist. If my experience with urologists is any indicator, you may have to insist that your urologist complete these tests PIOR to any treatment. In my case, the first 5 of the 6 urologists I worked with bypassed these tests and immediately proposed and started treatments. One of these 5 urologists referred me for pelvic floor physical therapy based on his guess that I may have had chronic pelvic floor pain and not chronic prostatitis. Three of them gave me prescriptions for antibiotics. The 5th one immediately performed a cystoscopy exam and scheduled me for Transurethral Resection of the Prostate or TURP prostate surgery, all without first testing to determine if I had an enlarged prostate. I canceled that appointment the following day. TURP prostate surgery is one of several common types of prostate surgery for men with an enlarged prostate or BPH. Prostate surgery is used for PBH, not for chronic prostatitis. Finally, three years and 5 urologists later, I saw with the 6th urologist. He, in stark contrast to the first five, immediately performed the urine flow and ultrasound of the prostate tests. At this point, I was well on my way to treating my chronic prostatitis with the Prostatitis 360 Protocol. The only reason I saw this 6th urologist was to finally rule out that prostate enlargement, such as early-stage enlargement, played a role in my chronic prostatitis symptoms.

If you have all the symptoms of chronic prostatitis discussed above and you have completed the tests in step one, I think you should insist on completing the three tests discussed below prior to starting any treatment.

Step Two: Initial Tests Done by Urologists

Chronic prostatitis is a complex condition that is difficult to diagnose. Diagnosis, however, is further complicated because, in many cases, urologists have a poor understanding of prostatitis and chronic prostatitis, fail to do the necessary testing, and often confuse the symptoms with other conditions. Many urologists fail to do even the minimum testing to rule out other common conditions with similar symptoms, confirm a diagnosis of prostatitis, and narrow it down to chronic prostatitis. There are three tests that your urologist must do to diagnose and properly treat chronic prostatitis. These three tests confirm or rule out BPH. BPH is the most common cause of symptoms similar to chronic prostatitis symptoms, and therefore, a critical step in diagnosing chronic prostatitis is to rule out our BPH.

   A. Bladder urine retention test. (often done by the primary care doctor prior to referral to a urologist) If the primary care doctor does not do it, it should be done by the urologist.
   B. A urine flow test is used to measure the strength of your urine flow.

CHAPTER 1
Understanding Chronic Prostatitis

C. Ultrasound of the prostate to measure the size of the prostate and determine if it's normal or enlarged.

These are simple, inexpensive, and routine tests, and most urologists have the equipment in their office to do a urine flow test and ultrasound of the prostate. These tests should be completed during

your initial visit with the urologist. The urologist should also do the bladder urine retention test if your primary care doctor did not complete it. If the urologist does not order or perform these tests, you should insist they be done either during the initial visit or the next scheduled visit. It is impossible to diagnose and properly treat chronic prostatitis without these tests. If the urine retention test, usually done by your primary care doctor, shows that you are fully emptying your bladder, it's the initial indicator that you don't have BPH, but you need the other two to truly rule out BPH. This is particularly important if you're over 50 because BPH is very common for men over 50.

Step Three: Advanced Tests Done by Urologists

Your urologist does the following tests primarily to more definitively rule out bacterial prostatitis, measure the level of inflammation, and determine if you have inflammatory (Type III A) or non-inflammatory (Type III B) chronic prostatitis.

A. EPS Test. This prostate fluid test, also known as the EPS or Expressed Prostate Secretions test, is done to test for white blood cells and cytokines in the prostate or seamon fluid, which are markers for infection and inflammation. In other words, whether you have inflammatory Type III A or non-inflammatory Type III B chronic prostatitis discussed above. Most men have non-inflammatory chronic prostatitis. This doesn't mean that there is no inflammation of the prostate. It just means that prostate fluid doesn't show the markers for inflammation.

B. Digital rectal exam or DRE. This exam is done by the urologist using a gloved finger to determine if the prostate is painful, tender, or sensitive when touched or rubbed by the doctor's gloved finger.

C. 4-Glass Test. This test has long been regarded as the gold standard for chronic prostatitis testing, but it's so cumbersome, time-consuming, and expensive that it's now rarely done anymore in the US. This test is designed to help determine if you have bacterial prostatitis or non-bacterial prostatitis and if you have inflammatory or non-inflammatory chronic prostatitis.

D. 2-Glass Test. The 2-glass test is an easier-to-administer replacement for the 4-glass test. Studies show it is almost as accurate (96%) as the 4-glass test.

E. Urine Tests. These tests are normally done earlier in the testing process (Step 1) by your primary care doctor, but they are sometimes repeated and expanded by urologists. Your urologist may order a mid-stream urine test if one was not done earlier. Another option is to analyze a full 24 or 48 hours of urine that is collected in a special container you take home with you. The mid-stream and 24/48-hour collection tests are intended to provide a more precise measurement of any difficult-to-detect bacterial infection.

F. A detailed inventory of your symptoms and symptom history. In Europe, urologists also ask patients to complete

CHAPTER 1
Understanding Chronic Prostatitis

the CPSS questionnaire. In the US, urologists are not aware of the questionnaire and don't use it. It's up to you to complete the CPSS questionnaire.

The tests discussed above are the standard battery of tests that should done by your primary care doctor and your urologist to rule out other conditions with similar symptoms and make a preliminary diagnosis of chronic prostatitis. There is no single test or combination of tests that will definitively confirm a diagnosis of chronic prostatitis. The best we can do today is to complete a careful inventory of the symptoms, do the battery of tests discussed above to rule out other conditions with similar symptoms and measure the types of inflammation that may indicate chronic prostatitis and to rule out other conditions with similar symptoms and measure the types of inflammation that may indicate chronic prostatitis.

Finally, there are two sets of tests discussed below that are not necessarily a part of the standard battery of tests that are done upfront to determine if you have chronic prostatitis. They are inflammation, blood tests, and rare conditions. The inflammation blood tests should be done after completing the standard battery of tests. The tests for rare conditions should be considered, if necessary, in the future if the treatment of the diet and supplement components of the prostatitis 360 protocol are not effective. Should these two sets of tests be Step 5 in a standard battery test? In an ideal world, they would be part of a complete battery of tests. The reality is that in many cases, it's a challenge to get primary care doctors, urologists, and insurance companies to do the tests that I have included in the four-step testing process. In fact, in my case, 4 of the 6 urologists I saw didn't do **any** testing and immediately prescribed various prescription drug treatments. I ultimately succeeded in getting most of these tests done, but only by being persistent with my doctors and health insurance providers. This book is a practical guide for men with chronic prostatitis and not an academic or theoretical discussion of all the testing tools for chronic prostatitis without regard to accessibility and cost.

Inflammation Blood Tests

The following are routine blood tests that your primary care doctor can order for you. Most health insurance plans will agree to provide these tests. These tests should be repeated once a year to measure any progress. These are important markers or indicators of chronic inflammation. The three tests are for C-reactive protein, Homocysteine, and Fibrinogen. When present above normal levels, they are indicators of what is known as Chronic Inflammatory Syndrome and are associated with an increased risk of heart disease and stroke. The standard reference range for C-reactive protein is up to 4.9 mg/L, but the optimal level is under 2 mg/L. the standard reference range for Homocysteine is up to 15 micromol, but the optimal level is under 10 micro/L. The standard reference range for Fibrinogen is under 460 mg/dl, but under 300 is ideal **(7)**

1. C-reactive Protein
2. Homocysteine
3. Fibrinogen

These three inflammation markers are not used to diagnose chronic prostatitis. However, once a diagnosis of chronic prostatitis has been established, these three inflammation markers can help you measure the level of inflammation in your body. If these inflammation markers are elevated, it does not mean that they are the cause of your chronic prostatitis, but there is growing scientific

CHAPTER 1
Understanding Chronic Prostatitis

evidence that they may be contributing factors to your chronic prostatitis symptoms. A 2017 study by Chen and colleagues, for example, found a link between high C-reactive protein levels and chronic prostatitis. **(8)**

There is a wide range of contributing factors that are believed to play a role in contributing to chronic prostatitis symptoms, including a highly inflammatory diet, a weak immune system, chronic stress, lack of aerobic exercise, and many more. We will address these and many other contributing factors to chronic prostatitis symptoms in the chapters that follow. These contributing factors may help us to understand the potential causes of the symptoms, but they do not represent the underlying cause or causes of chronic prostatitis. While some early scientific theories are being researched, science still does not understand the underlying causes of chronic prostatitis. If your levels of these inflammation markers are elevated, diet changes and supplements can help you manage these inflammation makers:

Fibrinogen: Elevated levels can be controlled with 180 mg (400iu) of vitamin E, nettle root extract, or daily dose of aspirin. Adding green tea(decaf) and garlic to your diet can also help. Nettle root extract is part of the Prostatitis 360 Protocol and may be a good starting point.

C-reactive Protein: Elevated levels can be controlled with high-quality DHA fish oil as part of a typical EPA / DHA fish oil supplement.

Homocysteine: High levels can typically be lowered with 800 mcg of Folate and 25 mcg of B-12 taken daily. Now Foods Folic Acid, with 800 mcg of folic acid and 25 mcg of B-12, is a good, widely available option.

Testing for Rare Conditions

The following are three rare conditions that cause symptoms similar to chronic prostatitis symptoms. These advanced tests should ideally be included in the battery of tests for men suffering from pain and urination symptoms of chronic prostatitis once they have completed the other tests. Unfortunately, the reality of the American healthcare system is that most Americans have health insurance provided by an HMO or PPO health insurance plan, and It's difficult to get this test.

1. Urethral Strictures

Urethral strictures are believed to affect approximately 1% of the male population and are twice as likely among men 65 and over. However, studies have been very limited, and the true prevalence is not well understood. Urethral strictures or physical obstructions in the urethra cause pain and urination symptoms. A retrograde urethrogram (RUH) test is used to determine whether you have urethral strictures. Urethral stricture is damage to the urethral tube that carries urine from the bladder through the prostate to your penis. If you have a urethral stricture, you may experience pain during urination, ongoing pain after urination, and partial blockage of urine flow. These symptoms mimic many of the symptoms of chronic prostatitis.

There are several challenges with testing for and treating urethral structures. The first is that health insurance companies in the US, whether you're in an HMO or PPO, will generally not pay for the test for urethral strictures. The test is not performed by a urologist. It is an outpatient test that typically must be performed in a hospital setting with specialized testing equipment. It is important to note that urethral strictures are

CHAPTER 1
Understanding Chronic Prostatitis

believed to be rare. The risk of overlooking a possible cause of your symptoms by not doing the test is low.

On the other hand, if nothing else works after trying diet, supplements, lifestyle changes, 5 mg Cialis, acupuncture, etc., testing for urethral strictures may be warranted, even if you must do it at your own expense. The test without insurance coverage is approximately $3,000. If, in fact, you have urethral strictures, surgery done by a urologist to remove them is generally safe and effective.

2. BPNO

Primary Bladder Neck Obstruction or BPNO is a physical blockage of the bladder neck at the start of the urethra and just above the prostate. It is believed to affect 3.9% to 7.6% of men. Serious chronic urination problems are the dominant symptoms of PBNO. Some pain and discomfort can also occur, but serious chronic urination problems are the dominant symptoms of the condition. In most cases, BPNO is not the cause of chronic prostatitis symptoms. There are tests called video urodynamic tests that can diagnose the condition, and both surgical and prescription drug treatments are available. If you are over 50 and your dominant symptoms are chronic serious urination problems, and you have not been tested for an enlarged prostate (BPH), it's important that you ask your urologist to test for an enlarged prostate because the system symptoms of BPH are very similar to PBNO. If you have both pain and serious urination symptoms and your symptoms have not improved after implementing the diet and supplement components of the Prostatitis 360 Protocol, you should work with your urologist to determine if you have PBNO.

3. Prostate Stones

Prostate stones, which are also known as prostate calculi, are small calcium deposits in the prostate. This condition is believed to be quite common, with 7% to 8% of men estimated to have prostatic calculi. Prostate stones are common among men over 40, and they are usually harmless. The most common symptoms are urination-related, including painful urination. Most men with prostatic calculi don't have symptoms, and the presence of the calculi stones is only discovered when testing for BPH. They can be surgically removed. If you're over 40 and your symptoms have not improved after implementing the diet and supplement components of the Prostatitis 360 Protocol, you should ask your urologist to do a prostate ultrasound to determine if you have prostate stones. This is a simple, inexpensive test covered by health insurance.

Measuring Chronic Prostatitis

The NIH CPSI

It is important at this stage to carefully inventory your symptoms, categorizing them as dominant (or primary), secondary, and by frequency and severity. Additionally, documenting the history and evolution of your symptoms is essential. Once a thorough and complete inventory of symptoms and symptom history has been compiled, two critical steps must be taken at this stage in the process.

The first step is a chronic prostatitis symptom evaluation, known as the Chronic Prostatitis Symptom Index (CPSI), developed by the National Institutes of Health (NIH) in the US. The CPSI is the global standard for measuring and scoring symptoms in men

CHAPTER 1
Understanding Chronic Prostatitis

with chronic prostatitis. Medical researchers around the world use it to assess and compare the benefits of various treatments for chronic prostatitis. It is absolutely critical for every man struggling with chronic prostatitis to complete the CPSI questionnaire and tabulate his score.

This is important whether you are just beginning to struggle with chronic prostatitis or if you've been living with it for several years and have not completed the questionnaire. Unfortunately, many men, like myself, may not even be aware of the existence of CPSI. This would not surprise me, as none of the six urologists I have seen in the past four years ever asked me to complete the CPSI or even mentioned the questionnaire's existence.

The chart below provides a breakdown of the CPSI by severity level. Pain is widely regarded as the most significant symptom, as it has the greatest impact on quality of life.

	Mild	Moderate	Severe
Pain:	0-7	8-13	14-21
Urination:	0-7	8-13	14-21
Q of L:	0-2	3-4	4-6
Total Score:	0-16	19-29	32-48

Once you complete the questionnaire, you can use this chart to determine the overall level of severity of your symptoms (total score) and your individual pain, urination, and quality of life severity scores. In my case, as an example, prior to starting the Prostatitis 360 Protocol, I had severe chronic prostatitis with a total score of 39 and a pain score of 17.

Below is the CPSI questionnaire. If you're struggling with chronic prostatitis, I recommend that you complete the questionnaire right now. Take the time to carefully read each question, answer it, and total your scores. You can also find a printable copy by doing an online search for "NIH CPSI questionnaire PDF."

NIH Chronic Prostatitis Symptom Index (NIH-CPSI)

Pain

1. In the last week, have you experienced any pain or discomfort in the following areas?

		Yes	No
a.	Between the rectum and testicles (perineum)	$\square_1$	$\square_0$
b.	Testicles	$\square_1$	$\square_0$
c.	Tip of the penis (not related to urination)	$\square_1$	$\square_0$
d.	Below your waist, in your pubic or bladder area	$\square_1$	$\square_0$

2. In the last week, have you experienced:

		Yes	No
a.	Pain or burning during urination?	$\square_1$	$\square_0$
b.	Pain or discomfort during or after sexual climax (ejaculation)?	$\square_1$	$\square_0$

CHAPTER 1
Understanding Chronic Prostatitis

3. How often have you had pain or discomfort in any of these areas over the last week?

    ❑$_0$ Never
    ❑$_1$ Rarely
    ❑$_2$ Sometimes
    ❑$_3$ Often
    ❑$_4$ Usually
    ❑$_5$ Always

4. Which number best describes your AVERAGE pain or discomfort on the days that you had it over the last week?

❑	❑ ❑ ❑ ❑ ❑ ❑ ❑ ❑ ❑ ❑
0	1 2 3 4 5 6 7 8 9 10
NO	EXTREME
PAIN	PAIN

Urination

5. How often have you had a sensation of not emptying your bladder completely after you finished urinating over the last week?

    ❑$_0$ Not at all
    ❑$_1$ Less than 1 time in 5
    ❑$_2$ Less than half the time
    ❑$_3$ About half the time
    ❑$_4$ More than half the time
    ❑$_5$ Almost always

6. How often have you had to urinate again less than two hours after you finished urinating over the last week?

❏0 Not at all ❏1 Less than 1 time in 5 ❏2 Less than half the time ❏3 About half the time   ❏4 More than half the time ❏5 Almost always Impact of Symptoms

7. How much have your symptoms kept you from doing the kinds of things you would usually do over the last week?

❏0 None ❏1 Only a little   ❏2 Some   ❏3 A lot

8. How much did you think about your symptoms over the last week?

❏0 None   ❏1 Only a little   ❏2 Some   ❏3 A lot

Quality of Life

9. If you were to spend the rest of your life with your symptoms just the way they have been during the last week, how would you feel about that?

❏0 Delighted ❏1 Pleased ❏2 Mostly satisfied ❏3 Mixed (about equally satisfied and dissatisfied) ❏4 Mostly dissatisfied ❏5 Unhappy ❏6 Terrible

Scoring the NIH-Chronic Prostatitis Symptom Index Domains

Pain: Total of items 1a, 1b, 1c,1d, 2a, 2b, 3, and 4 = _____

Urinary Symptoms: Total of items 5 and 6 = _____

CHAPTER 1
Understanding Chronic Prostatitis

Quality of Life Impact: Total of items 7, 8, and 9 = _____

Total overall score: Total of all items = _____

Name: _____

Date: _____

Why is the CPSI so important?

Every man suffering from chronic prostatitis (CP) should know their total score, as well as the separate domain scores for pain, urination, and quality of life. I recommend retaking the test and monitoring both the total and individual domain scores every six months, or whenever starting and completing a treatment protocol, or whenever there is a significant improvement or worsening of symptoms. The CPSI provides a baseline or reference point by which progress in treating chronic prostatitis can be measured.

Medical researchers around the world have used the CPSI for over 20 years to assess outcomes and success rates for chronic prostatitis treatments. I refer to the total and individual domain scores when discussing the scientific research results that I cite throughout the book to evaluate individual treatments for chronic prostatitis. A total score improvement greater than six is considered a "clinically significant" symptom improvement, which also indicates the effectiveness of the treatment being studied. The CPSI scores are crucial because they allow an individual to compare their score against the reported average improvement in the scores of patients in scientific studies related to a particular prostatitis treatment.

Another important questionnaire is the International Prostate Symptom Score (IPSS), which provides a more detailed, nuanced assessment of urination symptoms. It is universally used in benign prostatic hyperplasia (BPH) research and is also widely used in chronic prostatitis research. The IPSS uses a total score scale ranging from 0 to 35, where 0 to 7 indicates mild symptoms, 8 to 19 indicates moderate symptoms, and 20 to 35 indicates severe symptoms. There is also a separate quality of life score. You can download a printable version of the questionnaire online at ipss.pdf. I recommend that you complete this short questionnaire along with the CPSI.

Daily Health Diary

The next key step is to immediately begin a daily symptom and health diary. The importance of this step in the process of treating your prostatitis cannot be overstated. If you're struggling with prostatitis, you're flying a plane without an instrument panel if you don't maintain a detailed daily symptom and health diary. The only practical and effective way to maintain the diary is to use an electronic spreadsheet. Below is a simplified model of the basic design I use and recommend. I use a severity scale of 1 to 5, with 5 being very severe or poor for pain, sleep, etc.

A	B	C
Date	8/1/2021	8/2/2021
Pain – Dysuria (Scale: 1-5)	2	1.5

CHAPTER 1
Understanding Chronic Prostatitis

	1 am / 2.5 pm /	
Pain Overnight		
Pain Daytime	1.5 6 pm	1.5 am / 1 pm
Average (daytime)	2	1.5

Health – Indicators

Hours Slept	9:30 – 6	9:30 – 6
Sleep Quality (Scale of 1 to 5)	3.6	4
Stress Level	2.5	1.5
Headache (scale 1-5 & blank if none)		
Hemorrhoids		
Diarrhea / Constipation / Normal	D	N

Prescription - General

Atorvastatin (40mg)	1	Started: 1 x 40mg
Synthroid (125mcg.)	1	1

Prescriptions - Prostatitis

Flomax

Avodart

Cialis daily - 5mg

Supplements - Prostatitis

Pollen Extract (PollenAid® 500mg)	3	3
Saw Palmetto	2	2

Supplements - General

Vitamin E (400 IU)	1	1
Vitamin D (125mcg / 5000 IU)	3	3
Zinc (22mg / .05 Cooper)	1	1
Probiotics (Now 10 x 25 billion)	1	1

Lifestyle

Swim (min)	20	30
Weights (reps)	3 X 10	0
Standing Desk / Sit (Time - Hours)	8 / 6	7/7

Diet

Drinks
Water (cups)

Tea (Pepper Mint) (cups)

Wine

Breakfast
Eggs (#)

Bread - Gluten Free (slices)

Oatmeal (organic)

Shallots

Lunch

Dinner

CHAPTER 1
Understanding Chronic Prostatitis

This is the model for a daily prostatitis health diary. The purpose of the diary is to create a detailed daily record of your prostatitis symptoms, related health indicators, medications, supplements, lifestyle, diet, and any other factors that may directly or indirectly impact your symptoms. There is no one-size-fits-all format for the daily diary; each man suffering from prostatitis should adapt this basic model to his specific symptoms and other health indicators. Some men may need to track two or three different symptoms, along with their own set of health indicators, such as ongoing issues with acid reflux disease, ulcers, or high blood pressure. These are just a few examples of how the diary needs to be tailored to each man's specific symptoms and ongoing health issues. The diary is also the place to record any tests you take and the results.

    The diary functions as an electronic health record-keeping system. Column A contains the categories of information you're tracking, and Column B is always where you record the data for the current day. As you start a new day, you create a new column, and the data from Column B shifts to Column C, and so on, from day to day. This builds a history of your daily diary as you move across the spreadsheet. For anyone familiar with electronic spreadsheets from Microsoft, Apple, or Google, this is a very simple application. If you're new to spreadsheets, anyone reasonably familiar with them can help you set up your electronic diary. Most of the time, you'll just copy and paste most of the items from one day to the next, only updating the items that have changed, which makes it quick and easy to update and maintain your daily diary.

One key benefit that I want to emphasize at this point is the fact that the daily diary is perhaps the best—and possibly the only—effective way to monitor how each stage of the Prostatitis 360 Protocol, or any individual treatment, impacts your symptoms. For example, if you start the Prostatitis 360 diet or a supplement such as quercetin, you can monitor your symptoms daily and weekly to determine if and how much these individual treatments affect your symptoms.

This is where the daily diary becomes very powerful. In my case, for example, I know that the diet component of my treatment lowered my symptoms by 25% after six weeks, and it plateaued at a 30% improvement after eight to ten weeks. Another major improvement in my chronic prostatitis came from five supplements: pollen extract, the LESr version of saw palmetto, pumpkin seed oil, nettle root, and quercetin. Pollen extract and saw palmetto accounted for most of that improvement. What is very telling about these supplements is that I tried quercetin and flower pollen extract before implementing the diet. After 75 days, there was absolutely no improvement. In my case, any improvement that came from the various treatments I tried consistently began after 30 to 45 days.

The Prostatitis 360 Anti-Inflammation Diet resulted in approximately a 30% reduction in symptom severity and also laid the foundation that made it possible to achieve an additional 40% improvement from the five phytotherapy supplements mentioned above. My daily diary allowed me to understand what did and did not work in this situation and, most importantly, why. Over the past four years, I have tried over 30 different individual treatments, ranging from traditional medical treatments such as drugs and surgery to diet, supplements, and lifestyle changes. I have a detailed record of how each of those treatments did or did not

CHAPTER 1
Understanding Chronic Prostatitis

impact my chronic prostatitis. The daily diary has been the key to accurately measuring and evaluating what has worked. It has been the key tool for managing my chronic prostatitis treatment.

If you have completed all the evaluation, testing, and diagnosis steps in this chapter, you should now know if you have chronic prostatitis and the severity of your symptoms and have a system in place for tracking your condition going forward. The next step in the process is to understand the American healthcare system and the role of conventional medical care in treating chronic prostatitis.

CHAPTER 2
Chronic Prostatitis and the American Healthcare System

We now have a generation of men in the US who have needlessly struggled with chronic prostatitis. Millions of men could have benefited from dramatic, life-changing treatments for their condition if urologists in the US had begun incorporating diet and lifestyle changes, as well as supplements like flower pollen, quercetin, saw palmetto, nettle root, and pumpkin seed oil, into their practices for treating chronic prostatitis. Rigorous scientific research began emerging 35 to 40 years ago, demonstrating compelling evidence that these treatments can dramatically improve the symptoms of chronic prostatitis. These studies were widely published, discussed, and analyzed in major peer-reviewed urology journals in the US over the past 30 years.

Urologists and the urology community in the US acknowledged and admitted, and indeed often expressed frustration with their inability to help men with chronic prostatitis, especially given that one out of three patients visiting urologists had debilitating, often

CHAPTER 2
Chronic Prostatitis and the American Healthcare System

devastating, symptoms of chronic prostatitis. Yet, 30 years later, most urologists in the US have still not adopted these treatments. In fact, many urologists claim to have never even heard of these five supplements. This is in stark contrast to urologists in Europe, where saw palmetto, flower pollen, nettle root, and pumpkin seed oil have been incorporated into treatment plans for chronic prostatitis patients over the past 25 years.

Why have urologists in the US ignored what urologists in Europe widely adopted decades ago? To answer this question and address the broad range of issues it raises about the American healthcare system is not only far beyond the scope of this book, but it is also not directly relevant to the mission of this book or the Prostatitis 360 Protocol, which aims to help the millions of men in the US struggling with chronic prostatitis.

There are, however, some important aspects of the American healthcare system that every man in the US suffering from chronic prostatitis must understand to successfully manage the treatment of their condition. Men suffering from chronic prostatitis must understand the strengths and weaknesses of our healthcare system in general and how primary care doctors, urologists, and other specialists can and cannot help them.

Urologists in the US and the Treatment of Chronic Prostatitis

The following is an outline of the beliefs, attitudes, limitations, misconceptions, and misunderstandings about chronic prostatitis and how it is treated among many urologists in the US. In my interactions with nine different urologists from a wide range of practice types, I have encountered many of these traits:

⇒ The urologist who does not believe chronic prostatitis exists and only recognizes bacterial prostatitis and pelvic floor dysfunction.
⇒ The urologist who avoids any discussion of diagnosis or testing and simply begins writing prescriptions for commonly used drugs for BPH (benign prostatic hyperplasia), OAB (overactive bladder), and prostatitis.
⇒ The urologist who does not want to see you once you tell him that you've already tried TURP surgery and the commonly used prescription drugs.
⇒ The urologist who is convinced that prostatitis is a young man's disease and believes that if you're over 50, it's impossible for you to have chronic prostatitis.
⇒ The urologists who, if you're over 50, assume without doing any testing that you must have BPH and begin treating it by proposing TURP surgery and other treatments for BPH.
⇒ The urologist who has never heard of supplements or any other alternative treatments for chronic prostatitis.
⇒ The urologist who dismisses supplements as ineffective and potentially dangerous.
⇒ The urologist who does not review symptoms, perform any testing, or attempt any diagnosis and simply begins writing prescriptions.
⇒ The urologist who has never heard of the four types of prostatitis and refers to any form of prostatitis simply as "prostatitis."
⇒ The urologist who has never heard of the NIH Chronic Prostatitis Symptom Index (CPSI).

CHAPTER 2
Chronic Prostatitis and the American Healthcare System

⇒ The urologist who tells you that "chronic prostatitis is very difficult to treat," that he's never had any success treating it, writes a prescription, and clearly hopes you never return.

⇒ The urologist who becomes insulted if you discuss the scientific research you've done on chronic prostatitis or any alternative treatments such as supplements, seeing it as a challenge to his status as the expert in all things related to urology and the parent-child dynamic he has with his patients.

There are, of course, urologists in the US who do a thorough review of symptoms and symptom history, who do extensive testing, who understand the 4 types of prostatitis, who are familiar with supplements and other alternative treatments, and who are committed to treating chronic prostatitis in each his or her patients. Dr Daniel Shoskes at the Cleveland Clinic was not only a prominent chronic prostatitis researcher but also a practicing urologist who did careful symptom reviews, did extensive testing, and was familiar with and used supplements and other alternative treatments and more prior to his recent retirement. Another prominent chronic prostatitis researcher and practicing urologist is Dr J. Curtis Nickel at Queen's University in Canada, who has a very similar profile.

Dr Nichel created a list of six types of urologists in terms of their approach to chronic prostatitis. There are striking similarities between my experience with different urologists in terms of experience with urologists and the profiles created by Dr Nickel. His profiles of the different urologist types suggest that my experience was not unique, and it may reflect what many men find in their interactions with their urologists. The key glaring difference is that I never found the "committed urologist" described below.

The Nihilist - Doesn't believe prostatitis really exists as a disease entity, so doesn't have to see it or have to treat patients with it.

The Traditionalist - Prescribes antibiotics for those few patients in whom a positive uropathogen is cultured in the prostatic secretion and discharges the rest as having a nonurological problem.

The Antimicrobial Prescriber - Will prescribe antibiotics (independent of culture results, if one was ever done, one by one until he or she has prescribed all that are available. Then, he either starts all over or discharges the patient.

The Urodynamicist - Believes that symptoms due to subtle urinary obstruction that can only be evaluated and ameliorated by adhering to sound urodynamic principles.

The Interventionalist - Truly believes that all problems in the lower urinary tract can be dealt with by surgery. This urologist, a surgeon's surgeon, feels that once he has operated on the patient, there is nothing further he can do, and he therefore discharges the patient.

The Committed Urologist - Will use any and all investigations and potential beneficial treatments to help each individual patient. He does not abandon his patients but becomes frustrated with his impotence to deal with the majority of patients' very real complaints and concerns. **(1)**

There is no research in the US about the extent of urologists' knowledge about chronic prostatitis and how they diagnose and treat the condition. We can only speculate and use anecdotal data from personal experience to judge how many urologists fall into the

CHAPTER 2
Chronic Prostatitis and the American Healthcare System

categories or profiles outlined above. Dr Nickel's profile of the six types of urologists reflects his extensive experience working with urologists in Canada and the US. It's the most authoritative description we have of the traits and attitudes of urologists in treating chronic prostatitis. What it doesn't do is tell us what percentage of urologists in the US or Canada fall into the "Committed Urologist" category or the other categories. The situation in Europe is very different. While there's no extensive systematic research, there is significant scientific data that points to the extensive use by practicing urologists of a wide range of tests, the NIH CPSI, supplements, and more as part of comprehensive evaluation and treatment protocols. This is true not only in the major European countries such as Germany, France, and Italy but also in smaller countries with less sophisticated health care systems such as Greece. A 2020 survey of urologists in Italy and Greece compared how often they used 29 different diagnostic, lab, and clinical evaluation tools for their chronic prostatitis patients. The urologists in Greece and Italy commonly did a battery of 10 tests, and a significant percentage of the urologists in both countries did another 11. The evaluation tools commonly used included the CPSI and IPSS questionnaires, prostate ultrasound, two glass tests, digital rectal exam (DRE), and 5 more. In other words, urologists in Italy and Greece routinely invest time and effort in thoroughly evaluating their chronic prostatitis patients. **(2)** This is in stark contrast to the 6 urologists I saw in the US who, between them, performed a total of 4 tests, two of which were only done at my insistence.

Treating Chronic Prostatitis and Urology Care in the US: A Case Study

My personal experience with urologists and the urology care system in search of treatment for my chronic prostatitis serves as a valuable case study. Of course, this is the experience of just one man suffering from chronic prostatitis. It is not a comprehensive analysis of the entire healthcare system and how it manages chronic prostatitis. However, I believe it provides valuable insights and a reference point for other men struggling with chronic prostatitis. My experience includes a wide cross-section of healthcare systems in the US, including the two largest health insurance companies and the largest HMO in the country. I saw and worked with six urologists and had significant interactions with three more.

Appointments with doctors are typically limited to 20 or 30 minutes. This is a particularly serious problem for a complex condition like chronic prostatitis, which varies significantly from one individual to another. This was certainly my experience with all primary care doctors, urologists, and other specialists. The urologists I saw didn't have the time to conduct a careful evaluation of my symptom history or engage in a detailed discussion of testing and treatment options. None of the urologists I saw used detailed pre-appointment medical history and symptom questionnaires and none of them discussed, much less used, the NIH Chronic Prostatitis Symptom Index (CPSI) before or after the appointment. I believe administering the NIH evaluation questionnaires should be adopted as a standard part of treating BPH and prostatitis. This would be an especially effective use of pre-appointment evaluations for

CHAPTER 2
Chronic Prostatitis and the American Healthcare System

urologists who are limited by short appointment times due to HMOs and PPOs.

I saw six urologists during the first five years I struggled with chronic prostatitis and had significant interactions with three more. The nine urologists I saw represented a good cross-section of urologists in private practice as part of PPO networks, urologists who are part-time professors at a major research university medical system with one of the largest urology departments in the country, and urologists who are members of one of the largest urology practice groups in Southern California. None of these urologists had ever heard of, much less were familiar with, the use of supplements, diet, or any other alternative treatments, nor were they aware of conventional medical treatments such as UPOINT or shockwave therapy. All of them failed, except for the last one, to do the minimum basic testing necessary to rule out BPH and other similar conditions and confirm chronic prostatitis.

The first urologist did a cystoscopy exam and, without conducting any tests to determine whether I had an enlarged prostate, recommended TURP prostate surgery, which is designed for men with an enlarged prostate. The TURP surgery was completely ineffective. Unfortunately, this was early in my chronic prostatitis journey, and I had not yet done enough research to know that TURP surgery was intended for enlarged prostates, not for chronic prostatitis. One of the next urologists I saw, from the major medical research university and a part-time professor in urology, wanted to repeat the same process of doing a cystoscopy and recommending prostate surgery without conducting any tests to determine if I had an enlarged prostate. Fortunately, by this point, I had done enough research and I had enough personal experience with TURP surgery to know that it was ineffective for chronic prostatitis, and I declined his recommendation. When I pointed out that I had already had prostate surgery and it was unsuccessful, he argued that the urologist who performed the first surgery probably lacked extensive experience with TURP surgery, which he claimed was the reason for its failure.

In addition to antibiotics at the very beginning of the process, I tried at least one or two prescription drugs from each of the five major categories of prescription drugs commonly used by urologists in the US. None of them provided even minor improvement in my symptoms. One of the urologists I attempted to see, once he heard that I had already undergone prostate surgery and tried all the common prescription drugs, essentially told me there was nothing more he could do and recommended I work with a urologist affiliated with one of the major medical research universities.

The last and sixth urologist I saw, to his credit, performed the two key tests that the first five should have conducted. In fact, the first five urologists not only failed to perform the tests, but they didn't even discuss them. On my first visit to his office, this sixth urologist performed an ultrasound of my prostate to determine if it was enlarged, and he did a urine flow test to measure the strength of my urine flow. Based on those two tests and my previous testing history, he ruled out an enlarged prostate or BPH. By the time I saw this urologist, I was already well on my way to treating my chronic prostatitis. My primary goal in seeing a urologist at this point was to finally have the necessary tests done to rule out BPH as a possible contributing factor to my chronic prostatitis symptoms. Fortunately, I didn't need to request the tests they were, as they should be, part of the standard procedure in his office for men over 50 with pain and urinary symptoms.

Finally, years after I began my journey through the American healthcare system and nine urologists later, I had the testing I should have received the first time I saw a urologist—standard testing that

CHAPTER 2
Chronic Prostatitis and the American Healthcare System

all men with these symptoms should receive. However, when I told this sixth urologist that I believed I had chronic prostatitis, he insisted that it was impossible. He was absolutely convinced that I was too old to have chronic prostatitis because he firmly believed that only men under 40 could have the condition. He offered no alternative diagnosis but ruled out chronic prostatitis. Finally, like all the urologists I worked with, he was completely unfamiliar with diet, supplements, or any other alternative treatments for chronic prostatitis or BPH.

This was my odyssey through the traditional American healthcare system in search of treatment for chronic prostatitis in the second-largest metropolitan area in the US. This region includes four of the largest major medical university research systems in the US, with some of the most sophisticated urology departments in the country. While this is only the experience of one man struggling with chronic prostatitis, it serves as a case study and an example of the very limited ability of conventional healthcare, as practiced by most urologists, to treat chronic prostatitis.

If my experience is a reflection of the state of urology care for chronic prostatitis than most urologists in this country cannot help the millions of men suffering from chronic prostatitis, and this continues to have devastating consequences for most of those men. Yet the dominant healthcare model and mindset among men with chronic prostatitis remains stubbornly unchanged. Whether men have been struggling with chronic prostatitis for many years or have just begun to experience the symptoms, the prevailing belief remains firmly entrenched that if we have prostate or pelvic-related health issues, we turn to urologists, believing they are the experts in treating these conditions. This is part one of the belief system. The second part is that if these experts can't help us, there is no real alternative. This traditional conception of the role of the patient and the doctor, and the relationship between the two, still dominates urology and the American healthcare system in general.

Traditional and Alternative Healthcare in the US

One of the most disturbing aspects of the American healthcare system is how it is organized into adversarial camps between conventional medicine and alternative medicine. This is particularly evident in the adversarial attitude of traditional healthcare toward alternative medicine. In contrast, in Europe, what is referred to as alternative or CAM (complementary and alternative medicine) in the US is often an integrated part of the mainstream healthcare system in many European countries. Many European nations, led by Germany, have a long tradition of integrating scientifically proven supplements into mainstream healthcare. Supplements such as saw palmetto and flower pollen, which are scientifically proven, are classified as phytotherapy or nutraceuticals in Europe. These are manufactured by pharmaceutical companies and prescribed by doctors throughout the continent.

The overwhelming majority of primary care doctors and urologists in the US practice traditional or conventional medicine, which has proven to be largely ineffective in helping men suffering from chronic prostatitis. The alternative to this traditional healthcare is appropriately referred to as alternative medicine and is broadly known by various names, including integrative health, holistic health, CAM, or complementary and alternative medicine. Doctors who practice some form of alternative medicine are a small minority within the US healthcare system, and they operate

CHAPTER 2
Chronic Prostatitis and the American Healthcare System

largely outside what is covered by health insurance or available to members of HMOs or within PPO networks. Doctors specializing in treating the prostate or prostatitis within the alternative medicine field are an even smaller subset of this already limited group.

Why is this important for a man suffering from chronic prostatitis? Integrative health, or holistic health, is the multimodal healthcare model that most men with chronic prostatitis need in order to effectively manage and potentially cure their condition. The basic concept behind integrative, holistic health, or multimodal healthcare, is that it combines the best of all known and available treatment options, regardless of whether they are recognized as part of conventional healthcare or exist outside of it. Therefore, it incorporates a wide range of treatments, including diet, exercise, lifestyle changes, supplements, physical therapy, meditation, acupuncture, and any other proven treatment to address conditions like chronic prostatitis, alongside traditional healthcare for medical testing, pain management, and depression treatment.

Simply put, integrative health, in the case of chronic prostatitis, combines the necessary aspects of traditional medicine (like medical testing) and those that may help, such as physical therapy, acupuncture, and pain management, with a wide range of treatments that are not available through traditional medicine but have been scientifically proven to be effective in treating the condition. This approach is also known as a multimodal treatment model. A small percentage of men with chronic prostatitis may be treated with a single therapy, such as diet, a single supplement, or physical therapy, especially if their symptoms are mild. This single-treatment approach is known in the medical community as monotherapy. However, most men with moderate to severe symptoms will require a combination of treatments, known as multimodal treatment.

This is the heart of the problem for men suffering from chronic prostatitis in the US: conventional medicine, for the most part, doesn't work, and integrative or holistic medicine is, practically speaking, largely unavailable. Even when it is available, it's often not covered by health insurance, making it too expensive for most men. The answer I propose in this book is the Chronic Prostatitis 360 Protocol, which utilizes the integrative, holistic, multimodal treatment model.

The Limitations of Conventional Health Care in Treating Chronic Prostatitis

Perhaps the best way to understand the limitations of traditional healthcare when it comes to chronic prostatitis and the future of its treatment is to look at the history of an alternative protocol for heart disease. In the 1980s and 1990s, Dr. Ornish published groundbreaking research in peer-reviewed medical journals. In 1990, he published a highly influential book, which became a New York Times bestseller, with 1.5 million copies sold by 1996. The book discussed using diet, supplements, stress management, and lifestyle changes to treat heart disease, even advanced stages of heart disease. It took many years for the traditional medical community and doctors treating heart disease to gradually accept the Ornish diet program as a legitimate and effective approach. Eventually, the medical community acknowledged its validity, and Medicare and private health insurance companies began covering the Ornish program for heart disease patients.

Today, there are approximately 18 certified Ornish program treatment centers across 11 states offering a 9-week program, typically costing $9,500. Many of these centers are run by hospitals,

CHAPTER 2
Chronic Prostatitis and the American Healthcare System

and numerous health insurance companies, including Medicare, provide coverage for the program. Clearly, compared to the state of healthcare for chronic prostatitis treatment, the Ornish program for heart disease is light years ahead. However, the progress that the Ornish program has made in widespread adoption and availability has disturbing implications for the future of chronic prostatitis treatment in the US. The original research was conducted 40 years ago, and it has taken the past 20 years to see significant adoption and availability of the program. Despite this progress, the availability of the program remains severely limited. For example, California, the largest state in the country with 39 million people, has only two Ornish program locations.

To address this limitation, Dr. Ornish has introduced an online version of his program that provides near-universal access. However, most insurance companies do not cover the online program, limiting it to individuals who can afford it.

The Ornish program serves as a model for how to integrate a supplement/diet/lifestyle treatment program into the for-profit healthcare system in the US by monetizing it into a 9-week outpatient treatment that costs $9,500 and is covered by health insurance. While this model does not work for individual urologists in private practice, it is a potential solution for hospitals, large urology centers, or practice groups, who no longer have to choose between recommending a book and supplements at no profit or ignoring a proven treatment option. They can now provide a proven treatment program and generate the revenue necessary in a for-profit healthcare system.

The Ornish program is important as a case study because it illustrates that even when the traditional medical community accepts a new alternative supplement/diet/lifestyle treatment, a wide range of forces work to prevent the widespread adoption of that treatment program. This has certainly been the case with chronic prostatitis. However, there is one critical difference between treating heart disease and treating chronic prostatitis: conventional healthcare does have a range of treatments that are effective for heart disease, whereas conventional healthcare does not have effective treatments for chronic prostatitis. Heart disease patients and their doctors do not need to seek out alternative treatments, even if such treatments, like the Ornish program, are more effective without the use of drugs or surgery.

The Ornish case study raises an important question about the future of chronic prostatitis treatment in the US: Even if alternative treatments for chronic prostatitis are eventually accepted and recognized as effective by the mainstream medical system, will they be adopted, used, and made available to the vast majority of patients with HMO and PPO healthcare? In the final chapter, I address these and other related issues concerning the future of the Chronic Prostatitis 360 Protocol as a treatment for chronic prostatitis in the US.

Health Insurance and Chronic Prostatitis Treatment in the US

This book is a practical guide for the vast majority of men in the US who have some form of HMO or PPO health insurance, which accounts for 92% of all Americans with private health insurance as well as the many men in the US who lack health insurance. Unlike the small number of individuals with Point of Service (POS) health insurance, which allows them the freedom to see any doctor in any specialty anywhere in the US, the vast majority of Americans with HMO and PPO plans have a wide range of restrictions and

CHAPTER 2
Chronic Prostatitis and the American Healthcare System

limitations on their access to healthcare. These limitations have important consequences for healthcare in general and for men suffering from chronic prostatitis in particular. These health plans impose limits on healthcare for chronic prostatitis, which have profound implications for men struggling with this condition.

The limitations and constraints of PPO and HMO healthcare make it virtually impossible to treat chronic prostatitis effectively. Going outside the PPO or HMO networks for doctors and approved treatments and tests is, for most men, prohibitively expensive.

A Case Study: Chronic Prostatitis and Health Insurance

My experience with the health insurance system illustrates many of the challenges in treating chronic prostatitis in the US. My experience with the largest HMO in the US is an example of the limits on access to specialists and the challenges posed by short appointments with doctors. In this case, I never actually saw a urologist. My primary care provider at the HMO did enough initial testing to warrant seeing a urologist but was unable, following the HMO's guidelines, to refer me to one. Instead, I was forced to see a urology nurse. The urology nurse, without conducting any tests or a thorough review of my symptoms, prescribed Flomax, which not only did not work but actually worsened my symptoms. My 20-minute appointments with my primary care doctor and the urology nurse were simply too short to properly evaluate a complex condition such as chronic prostatitis.

My experience with the largest health insurance company in the US, which provides PPO health plans, highlights some of the other challenges of specialized urology care. Despite a referral from a urologist within the PPO network for a urethral stricture test, the PPO plan refused to cover the test—even after an appeal. Performing the procedure to remove urethral strictures, if necessary, was also out of the question. I encountered the same issue with short appointment times with the six urologists I saw through two different health insurance companies and their PPO plans. My appointments were typically limited to 20 minutes, which made it impossible to conduct the careful evaluation necessary for a complex condition like chronic prostatitis.

The Status of Alternative Treatments for Chronic Prostatitis

The American healthcare system, in the broadest sense, has failed men with chronic prostatitis. Conventional healthcare has proven ineffective in treating chronic prostatitis, and many men with the condition lack the information they need about alternative treatments. Men suffering from chronic prostatitis need to go through a process that can be summed up as knowledge, belief, and determination. They need information about alternative treatments, and that information must be presented as credible to instill the belief and confidence necessary to take action. Only then can they summon the will and determination to implement these alternative treatments.

Some men with prostate health problems do turn to supplements in search of alternative treatments. However, most of these men have BPH (benign prostatic hyperplasia) or BPH-related urinary symptoms. One study found that 30% of men with prostate health problems in the US have experimented with or are currently using over-the-counter supplements, which means 70% are not using supplements, the single best category of alternative treatments for chronic prostatitis. Moreover, it is unclear whether the 30% using supplements are taking the three proven supplements rather than the over 200 "prostate health" supplements

CHAPTER 2
Chronic Prostatitis and the American Healthcare System

available, many of which, if they do contain one of the five proven supplements, typically include it in a dosage too low to be effective.

A key part of the problem is that men in the US live in an information desert when it comes to alternative treatments for chronic prostatitis. Online forums, chat groups, and Facebook pages are filled with thousands of men discussing their struggles with chronic prostatitis. While these discussions are anecdotal and not scientifically valid, they provide valuable insights into the prevailing thinking among individuals suffering with prostatitis. Two common themes emerge in these online discussions: one is the recurring story of men who have suffered for years with prostatitis and have seen numerous urologists, often with no cure in sight. A paraphrased example might read, "I have been struggling with prostatitis for over 10 years, seen more than 20 urologists, and I'm at the end of my rope." Another common theme is members comparing notes about the antibiotics recommended by their urologists and discussing which works best. In several years of following these forums, I have yet to find any reference to proven treatments such as quercetin, pollen extract, saw palmetto, nettle root, or pumpkin seed oil.

Information about alternative treatments for chronic prostatitis remains scarce and very limited. The most widely available and accessible health information online offers little or no guidance on alternative treatments for the general reader. Even respected health sources such as the Cleveland Clinic, the Mayo Clinic, Harvard Health, and the Urology Care Foundation provide minimal information on alternative treatments. For example, the Cleveland Clinic briefly mentions quercetin and pollen but makes no reference to diet or other lifestyle changes. The Mayo Clinic discusses the three most common diet changes—alcohol, caffeine, and spicy foods—and suggests these should be "limited" rather than eliminated. It also references pollen but cautions against the use of supplements in general. The Urology Care Foundation, part of the American Urological Association, mentions reducing alcohol, caffeine, and spicy foods, as well as consuming less sugar. However, their statement about supplements is misleading:

> "Unfortunately, supplements have not helped when tested in medical studies. There was no evidence that herbs and supplements improve prostatitis. Options that have been tried and failed to help prostatitis include ryegrass pollen, a chemical found in green tea and onions, and saw palmetto extract. Supplements can affect other treatments, so if you want to try herbal supplements, please tell your doctor first."

The reference to the "chemical found in green tea and onions" is likely quercetin. This statement from the largest and most respected urology association in the US is inaccurate. The three supplements it references have, in fact, been proven effective in rigorous scientific studies. It is false that they have been "tried and failed" in treating chronic prostatitis. In reality, several studies and meta-analyses published in the official journals of the American Urological Association have reported improvements in chronic prostatitis symptoms ranging from 70% to 96%. This is vastly superior to the typical 30% improvement from many of the drugs prescribed by urologists, many of whom are members of the American Urological Association. This represents a case where urologists in the US are unable to help men with chronic prostatitis, and the association representing them actively discourages the very alternative treatments these men need.

CHAPTER 2
Chronic Prostatitis and the American Healthcare System

The best and most authoritative information on alternative treatments comes from the National Institutes of Health (NIH) website, which lists quercetin, pollen, and saw palmetto and uses the term "phytotherapy" to describe these supplements, acknowledging them as recognized treatments for chronic prostatitis. It also recommends the use of the NIH Chronic Prostatitis Symptom Index (CPSI) questionnaire to evaluate the severity of individual chronic prostatitis cases. This stands in stark contrast to the American Urological Association, which leads and represents urologists and the urology community in the US. Websites like WebMD and Healthline also offer limited information on alternative treatments for chronic prostatitis, and the Wikipedia page on chronic prostatitis completely ignores alternative treatments, focusing only on traditional urological treatments.

Not only do these common and respected sources of information on chronic prostatitis focus almost entirely on conventional medical treatments, but the information on alternative treatments is either too limited to be useful or, in some cases, distorted and inaccurate, which may discourage men from seriously considering these alternatives. None of these websites reference the research done on the effectiveness of diet, lifestyle changes, and supplements. The majority of information on these sites is still dedicated to traditional urology treatments, and references to alternative treatments are extremely limited. The Wikipedia page on chronic prostatitis is entirely focused on traditional treatments, while 40 years of published, rigorous scientific research on proven treatments for chronic prostatitis is completely ignored.

The information about alternative treatments is readily available online and free of charge, but it requires a deeper level of research, typically found in major urology journals in the US, Europe, and around the world. These journals contain summaries of original research trials and scientifically proven, trusted information. However, this level of research is not easily accessible to most individuals outside of the medical field. While much of this research is published in English, it often uses medical, scientific, and research terminology that can be difficult to understand at first, but with some time, effort, and determination, it is possible to make sense of this medical journal information. We need an information revolution in the US to make alternative treatment options for chronic prostatitis more widely available. This book was written to help lead that information revolution.

A New Patient-Driven Healthcare Model

We also need a new healthcare model in the US for men with chronic prostatitis, with a radical shift—a paradigm shift—in the role of the patient, the role of the doctor, and the conventional healthcare system in treating this condition. Men with chronic prostatitis need to recognize the very limited ability of most urologists to help them and rethink how they take ownership of their chronic prostatitis treatment. Under this new, patient-centric, patient-led model, we integrate the urologist, primary care doctor, medical specialists, and the healthcare system as a whole with a range of scientifically proven alternative treatments to create an integrated, holistic, multimodal chronic prostatitis treatment program. This program would be customized for and led by each individual suffering from chronic prostatitis. The conventional American healthcare system will not adapt to meet the needs of men with chronic prostatitis. The responsibility falls on each man suffering from chronic prostatitis to change their attitude and approach to both the traditional healthcare system and alternative treatments for their condition.

CHAPTER 2
Chronic Prostatitis and the American Healthcare System

Change is difficult under the best of circumstances, but a dramatic shift in beliefs and attitudes is particularly challenging. The key first step is creating awareness that there are proven alternatives for treating chronic prostatitis. Men suffering from chronic prostatitis have powerful incentives to change if they understand the alternatives available to them. That is the mission of this book and the Prostatitis 360 Protocol: to provide men suffering from chronic prostatitis with the information, resources, and tools to treat this devastating condition.

The Role of Conventional Medical Care

Conventional medical care does not play a direct role in the treatment of chronic prostatitis, but it plays an important role in helping men with chronic prostatitis manage their condition and treat some secondary side effects. Treatments such as physical therapy for chronic pelvic floor dysfunction, erectile dysfunction (ED), depression, acupuncture for pain management, daily 5 mg Cialis, Botox, and addressing the impact of health conditions such as diabetes, ulcers, and irritable bowel syndrome are all integral and important parts of the Chronic Prostatitis 360 Protocol. These treatments are discussed in detail in the chapters that follow, with Chapters 9 and 10 dedicated to treating ED and depression. Conventional medical treatments are the primary treatments for these two common side effects of chronic prostatitis.

CHAPTER 3
Conventional Medical Treatment for Chronic Prostatitis

In the US, the established, widely used conventional medical treatments for chronic prostatitis have been proven to be ineffective. However, there are new and emerging conventional medical treatments that are not widely known or used that have been proven to be effective today or may emerge as potential treatment options in the future. Some of these treatments are recommended options as part of the Chronic Prostatitis 360 Protocol, including 5mg daily Cialis and acupuncture. Others are potential future treatments if they become widely available, covered by insurance, and proven by additional rigorous scientific research.

Prescription Drugs for Chronic Prostatitis

Prescription drugs are the most common conventional medical treatments used by urologists in the US to treat chronic prostatitis.

CHAPTER 3
Conventional Medical Treatment for Chronic Prostatitis

There are two broad categories of drugs used by urologists to treat chronic prostatitis. The first category is antibiotics. Here, the scientific evidence is overwhelming that antibiotics do not work and can actually make the condition worse. Despite this overwhelming scientific evidence, urologists continue to prescribe antibiotics. Antibiotics don't work because they're designed for bacterial infections and chronic prostatitis, which is a nonbacterial condition. Men with chronic prostatitis should avoid antibiotics because they can damage your overall gastrointestinal or gut health and undermine your body's ability to fight inflammation, including inflammation of the prostate.

The other broad category of drugs is five classes of drugs developed to treat BPH, overactive bladder, and erectile dysfunction that are also used to treat chronic prostatitis. The following is a list of the five major classes of these prescription drugs. All of the drugs in all five classes of drugs are designed in one way or another to either lower inflammation and relax the prostate, bladder, and/or surrounding tissue or treat erectile dysfunction.

Class of Drug Generic & Brand Names

1. **Alpha 1 blocker**   A. Terazosin / Hytric
   B. Alfuosin / Uroxanddra   C. Doxazosin / Cardura
   D. Silodosin / Rapaflo   E. Tamsulosin / Flomax

2. **5 alpha-reductase inhibitors**
   Block the conversion of testosterone to DHT. FDA-approved
   A. Finasteride / Proscar
   B. Dutasteride / Avodart

3. **Anticholinergic agent**
    Relaxes bladder smooth muscle. FDA approved to treat
    A. Oxybutynin / Oxytro
    B. Fesoterodine / Tovia
    C. Darifenacin / Tovia
    D. Tolterodine Tartrate / Detrol LA

4. **Beta-3 adrenergic agonist**
    Increases bladder capacity by relaxing bladder muscles. FDA approved for overactive bladder
    A. Mirabegron / Myrbetriq

5. **PDE 5 inhibitors**
    Promotes smooth muscle relaxation of the prostate, bladder and surrounding areas. FDA approved for erectile dysfunction
    A. Tadalafil / Cialis
    B. Sildenafil / Viagra

These are the five most common classes of prescription drugs used in the US to treat chronic prostatitis. For each class, I include a partial list of some of the most common prescription drugs in each class used for chronic prostatitis.

They continue to be widely used by urologists despite the fact that years of experience and extensive scientific research using randomized placebo-controlled scientific studies consistently show that four of these five classes of drugs do no better than a placebo or a 30% improvement in symptoms. Medical researchers and the scientific community regard an improvement of greater than 25% to 30% as the minimum standard for treatment to even begin to be considered potentially effective, and typically, a 40% improvement is considered the threshold for success.

In a study done by Nickel, 12 alpha-blockers are compared to quercetin for the treatment of prostatitis. Alpha-blockers are the only

CHAPTER 3
Conventional Medical Treatment for Chronic Prostatitis

class of drugs that has done better than 30%, and for most drugs in this class, the percentage of improvement is just above 30%. The comparable percentage for quercetin, on the other hand, was 67%. Alfuzosin is the only drug that has exceeded the 50% threshold and attained 60% improvement. Studies of Alfuzosin, however, are mixed. A 6-month study of 4857 men found that only 20% had a significant improvement.**(1)** All of these drugs, including Alfuzosin, have serious potential side effects. Many patients discontinue these drugs due to side effects. None of these drugs, including Alfuzosin, matched the effectiveness of the five proven chronic prostatitis supplements. All of which have consistently demonstrated symptom improvement of 70% or better with minor or no side effects.

Daily 5mg Cialis: A Safe and Effective Conventional Drug Treatment

The only conventional medical drug treatment that has been proven to be safe and provide greater than 70% improvement in chronic prostatitis symptoms, if used long term, is daily 5mg Cialis in the PDE 5 class of drugs. Several recent studies using 5mg daily Cialis for a minimum of 3 months and normally requiring 6 months or more have proven in RCT studies to be effective.

Cialis Research

During the past five years, there have been 7 RCT studies of 5 mg Cialis for the treatment of chronic prostatitis. Many of these studies were short, lasting from 4 to 6 weeks. All the studies reported significant improvement in total CPSI scores as well as pain, urination, and quality of life scores. Unfortunately, there appear to have been no studies of 10, 15, or 20 milligrams of daily use of

Cialis. A meta-analysis done by Alzahrani and colleagues in 2022 of seven RCT studies with 584 patients reported significant reductions in total CPSI scores as well as pain, urination, and quality of life scores. **(2)** A 6-week 2022 study by Tawfik and colleagues with 140 patients reported that 50.8% of the Cialis group had a 25% or greater reduction in total CPSI scores compared to just 5.4% for the placebo group. Urination and quality of life scores improved significantly, but the pain score remained unchanged in the Cialis group.**(3)** Another six-week study (Park 2019) also reported improvements in all areas except the pain score. However, three-month studies (Pirola 2020, Anas 2023) report improvement in total CPSI scores, urination, quality of life as well as pain scores. The 3-month 2023 Anas study reported that 79.6% of the patients had a substantial improvement in CPSI scores, including the pain score, as well as a substantial improvement in the ED score. **(4)** While the number of studies and the number of patients studied is limited, there are two preliminary conclusions we can draw from these studies. The first is that 5mg Cialis can provide significant improvement in chronic prostatitis symptoms, including pain symptoms if taken for three or more months. The second is that Cialis has the advantage of improving both chronic prostatitis and erectile dysfunction (ED) symptoms.

There is one long-term study, however, that suggests that Cialis can provide substantial improvement if taken for over a year. A 2019 study by Pinault and colleagues involved 25 patients who took Cialis for 15 months. The results in this study were very impressive, with 19 or 76% of the patients reporting a significant improvement or better, including 11 with substantial improvements and 7 with dramatic improvements, which came close to providing a cure for some of the seven patients. **(5)** Unfortunately, this is just one study with only 25 patients. If, in the future, there are more studies

CHAPTER 3
Conventional Medical Treatment for Chronic Prostatitis

involving a larger number of patients, Cialis could emerge as a treatment comparable to saw palmetto or perhaps even flower pollen if you take it for longer than 6 months. One study compared Cialis with flower pollen. The three-month study by Matsukawa and colleagues done in 2020 with 100 patients compared Cialis and Cernilton flower pollen. While both groups reported improvement, the pollen extract group reported that 50% of the patients had a 50% or greater improvement in their symptoms compared to just 8.9% for the Cialis group.**(6)** It's important to note that, unlike the five main chronic prostatitis phytotherapy, Cialis requires 6 months or more to see the full benefit. However, it has the important advantage of helping with erectile dysfunction. Therefore, adding Cialis to the five core phytotherapies may be a good strategy for men with ED. But even if you don't have ED, Cialis may complement your phytotherapy treatment program because researchers believe that it improves the symptoms of chronic prostatitis in ways that are different from the five phytotherapies. The key difference between Cialis and the phytotherapies is that Cialis is a drug and has a greater potential for side effects. Studies show that in most cases, side effects are rare and minor, but there is the potential for more serious side effects. It's important to carefully monitor Cialis for side effects, especially if you use it long-term. The side effects of Cialis are minor compared to other major prescription drugs used to treat chronic prostatitis, all of which have potentially serious side effects and are often discontinued by patients due to their side effects. Cialis is the only prescription drug that has been proven to be safe and effective in significantly reducing the symptoms of chronic prostatitis if taken for one year or more.

Despite the fact that Cialis is the only safe and effective prescription drug for chronic prostatitis, most urologists in the US are not familiar with Cialis as a treatment for chronic prostatitis and don't prescribe it. None of the 6 urologists I saw discussed much less prescribed Cialis as a treatment for chronic prostatitis. The best option may be to simply ask your primary care doctor for a prescription for Cialis. It's important to keep in mind that Cialis is a long-term treatment. It may take three months to see significant benefits, especially in your pain symptoms, and it may take 6 to 12 months or more before you see the full benefit of Cialis.

The five primary supplements recommended in the Prostatitis 360 Protocol have much more extensive scientific research, begin to work faster and achieve better overall results than Cialis. Nevertheless, I believe Cialis can complement the treatment options for men with chronic prostatitis. Cialis is part of the chronic Prostatitis 360 Protocol as an add-on treatment to the five primary supplements for chronic prostatitis for all men, especially for men with erectile dysfunction. I discuss Cialis in additional detail as a treatment for ED in chapter 9, which is dedicated to sexual health for men with chronic prostatitis.

Acupuncture

Acupuncture has gained widespread acceptance by medical establishments in the US over the past 10 years as a scientifically proven and effective treatment for several medical conditions. Studies show that it is also effective for treating chronic prostatitis pain. It is effective in treating pain but not the other symptoms of chronic prostatitis, such as urination symptoms, and it works for many, but not all, men with chronic prostatitis.

A 2023 meta-analysis of 17 studies, including RCT studies with 1,455 patients, reported significantly lower pain using both the CPSI and the VAS measures of pain. **(10)** Meta-analyses such as this that include RCT studies provide the strongest scientific validation of the

CHAPTER 3
Conventional Medical Treatment for Chronic Prostatitis

effectiveness of medical treatments. Some individual studies have reported that it is typically effective in about 60% of patients and that the improvement in chronic pain ranges from 30% to approximately 50% when it works. Some studies have also looked at whether the benefits last beyond the initial treatment and have reported that they do. A 2021 study of men with chronic prostatitis involved 20 sessions over 8 weeks and reported that 60.6% of the patients had a significant reduction in pain of at least 6 points on the CPSI pain scale. This study was particularly interesting because it included a 24-week follow-up to determine whether these pain reductions were lasting. The reduction in pain after 24 weeks remained unchanged.**(11)** A study of 100 patients with chronic prostatitis over a 24-week period reported a response rate of 92% and, on average, a 50% reduction in pain.**(12)** Acupuncture has clear benefits and clear limitations. It doesn't work for all men, and the benefits are limited to reducing pain by approximately 50%. It doesn't help with the other symptoms of chronic prostatitis. However, among conventional medical treatments, acupuncture has a very important advantage because there are no side effects. It is also relatively inexpensive, and in many cases, PPO and HMO health plans will pay for a basic course of treatment of 10 sessions over 8 to 10 weeks. This may not be adequate because many successful studies involve 20 sessions over 8 to 10 weeks. Many doctors specializing in pain medicine and pain clinics often include an acupuncturist on staff that focuses on treating pain as part of the practice. If you're part of a PPO, look for an in-network pain specialist or clinic that has an acupuncturist on staff. This may be the easiest way to get health insurance companies to approve and pay for acupuncture treatments.

Cialis, acupuncture, the treatment of severe depression, which is discussed in Chapter 10, and initial and ongoing chronic prostatitis testing are some important ways that conventional medicine can help men with chronic prostatitis. There are some additional treatments available through a limited number of urologists with specialized training and medical equipment. These are proven to be effective in a small number of rigorously scientific studies. Very few urologists are familiar with much less have the training and in some of these treatments the specialized medical equipment to offer these treatments. They exist, but in practical terms, they are not accessible options for most men with chronic prostatitis. This book is not a theoretical or academic study of chronic prostatitis. Rather, it's a practical guide intended to be easily accessible to all men with chronic prostatitis, with a particular focus on the 92% of men in the US who obtain their healthcare through HMOs and PPOs. Therefore, I provide only brief descriptions of each of these treatments largely for future reference until and if they become more widely available. These include the UPOINT system, Botox, prostate massage, and shockwave therapy.

New, Emerging, and Potential Future Treatments

The UPOINT System

The UPOINT System is not a new treatment but a new multimodal treatment model similar in concept to the chronic Prostatitis 360 Protocol. However, unlike the Prostatitis 360 Protocol, UPOINT is almost entirely limited to conventional medical treatment options with one critical exception. When Dr. Shoskes and others first introduced it in the early 2000s, it incorporated the use of quercetin, flower pollen, and saw palmetto. However, many more recent descriptions of this system have removed references to supplements

CHAPTER 3
Conventional Medical Treatment for Chronic Prostatitis

as a treatment option. The protocol calls for an extensive battery of medical tests as part of the process of selecting the best treatment options. However, those treatment options do not include what I believe is critical to successfully treating chronic prostatitis, such as diet and lifestyle changes, as well as all five proven supplements. The multimodal approach is the right approach, but UPOINT doesn't go nearly far enough and continues to rely on conventional medical treatments that have proven to be largely ineffective. The extensive battery of medical tests required by UPOINT is what all men with chronic prostatitis should have available, but again, in practical terms, it's an open question if our HMO and PPO-based healthcare will ever agree and pay for this battery of tests.

UPOINT System Research

A review of studies done by Bryk and colleagues in 2021 found a reduction of six points or greater that ranged from 84% to 75% for three of the studies, and the fourth study done by Krakhotkan in 2019 reported an average improvement that ranged from 13.9% to 29.8%. This study used 1000 mg of quercetin and only 63 mg of Cernilton. **(7)** All these studies used some combination of quercetin, flower pollen, and saw palmetto, which may explain why the results were promising. The first study was the only study to show results comparable to those of flower pollen and saw palmetto. The other studies were comparable to quercetin. In fact, the first study, which showed an 84% improvement, was done by Shoskes and colleagues in 2010 and reported that flower pollen and quercetin provided the single most effective treatment among the treatments used in the study. If, in the future, the UPOINT system incorporates diet, lifestyle, and the other components of the Prostatitis 360 Protocol, it could become a platform for the adoption of the Prostatitis 360

Protocol by the urology establishment in the US and around the world. I believe that this is the real potential value of the UPOINT System.

Botox Prostate Injections

Research done during the past 15 years on the use of Botox to treat men with chronic prostatitis has been very promising, particularly in treating the pain symptoms of the condition. It has also been used with some success to treat BPH, IC/Painful Bladder Syndrome, and Overactive Bladder. A 2019 meta-analysis of Botox injections for chronic prostatitis involving six studies, including RCT studies and 283 patients, reported a significant decrease in pain as well as some improvement in the urination symptoms in some of the studies. Most of the studies used 200 units of Botox injected into the prostate and tracked the outcomes for six months. **(8)**

A 2015 RCT study with 60 men included in the meta-analysis reported an impressive reduction in pain symptoms that remained consistent during the six-month follow-up period. In the study, 79.9% of the patients reported a 10-point or greater reduction in overall CPSI scores, and 82.1% of the patients reported an 8-point or greater reduction in pain on the VAS pain scale. **(9)** These results are very impressive both in terms of the extent of pain reduction and the higher percentage of patients who benefited. As a monotherapy, these results are comparable to studies of flower pollen and saw palmetto as a monotherapy treatment for chronic prostatitis pain but not urination symptoms. Flower pollen and saw palmetto remain superior treatments because they reduce both pain and urination symptoms. Several other issues with Botox make it less attractive than flower pollen or saw palmetto as a treatment option. One of the studies in the meta-analysis tracked patient outcomes for 12 months and reported a drop off in pain reduction after 9 months. This means

CHAPTER 3
Conventional Medical Treatment for Chronic Prostatitis

that Botox treatment may need to be repeated every 9 to 12 months to be effective. A single 200-unit Botox injection course of treatment is very expensive and may need to be repeated. Botox treatment for chronic prostatitis is not covered by health insurance. It may be difficult to find doctors with experience doing Botox injections for chronic prostatitis. Therefore, Botox injections as a treatment for chronic prostatitis may only be a viable option for men who can afford it and who have seen some benefit but have not attained a 50% or greater reduction in pain symptoms after implementing the complete Prostatitis 360 Protocol.

Prostate Massage

Prostate massage is typically a 10-week program of weekly treatments similar to UPOINT in that it is rarely practiced in the US and is not widely available. It was widely used in Europe in the first half of the 20th Century and is still one of the most common treatments for chronic prostatitis in several countries, including Russia, Turkey, and China. A 2008 survey of urologists in China found that 54% recommend prostate massage for chronic prostatitis patients. It requires training in proper massage techniques that is not readily available to urologists in the US. There have been some small studies in the US, including a 1999 UCLA study by Shoskes that showed promise, but 19% of the men who initially benefited saw a recurrence of their symptoms after the study was completed. Many studies, including a 2008 meta-analysis by Mishra and a 2006 study by Ateya, reported no benefit. The key issue with the prostate message may be the extent and quality of the training in proper prostate massage techniques for urologists. When the prostate massage was widely practiced in Europe during the first half of the 20th century, urologists completed extensive training in proper prostate massage techniques. In fact, there was an institute in Stockholm, Sweden, dedicated to training urologists in prostate massage. It attracted urologists from throughout Europe as well as some from North America.

Shockwave Therapy

Shockwave therapy is another treatment possibility that has been studied largely by medical researchers and has shown promise in a very limited number of scientific studies as a treatment for chronic prostatitis. There are several versions of shockwave therapy, including LIST, low-intensity shockwave therapy, and EWST, or extra corporal shockwave therapy. These treatments require special equipment, and again, very few urologists are familiar with these treatments or have the training and equipment to provide these therapies. If they become widely available and are proven in a larger number of scientific studies to be effective, they would be particularly interesting because shockwave treatments focus on pain and appear to have their greatest success in reducing pain. Chapter 6, which focuses on pain, provides additional information on shockwave therapy.

Minimally Invasive Surgery

Finally, a new class of less invasive and minimally invasive surgical treatments for BPH, including Rezum and Urolift ™, has been scientifically studied and shown promising results in treating the urinary and pain symptoms associated with BPH. These new treatments for BPH require specialized training and equipment, and a growing number of urologists have received this training largely in major metropolitan areas. They have not been studied as a treatment for chronic prostatitis, but some urologists claim, despite the lack of scientific evidence, that these less invasive treatments

CHAPTER 3
Conventional Medical Treatment for Chronic Prostatitis

can potentially help chronic prostatitis patients. If, in the future, scientific studies are done to demonstrate these treatments can be effective for men with chronic prostatitis, they may emerge as additional treatment options. The open question is if existing surgery options for BPH have not been effective in treating chronic prostatitis, why would these new, less invasive surgery options necessarily be any different? Therefore, I believe a great deal of caution is warranted until clear scientific evidence proves that these new, less invasive surgical treatments are, in fact, effective. This is especially true because urologists, as I know from personal experience, have promoted and continued in some cases to promote surgery designed for BPH as a treatment for chronic prostatitis when it has been consistently proven that it is not effective.

Summary of the role of conventional medicine in treating chronic prostatitis

The following is a summary of the role of conventional medicine in treating chronic prostatitis organized by urologists, primary care doctors, and other specialists:

Urologists
1. The initial chronic prostatitis medical testing and ongoing testing and monitoring.
2. Prescription for Cialis. In many cases, your primary care doctor can also provide you with a prescription for five mg daily Cialis.
3. Treatment for ED or erectile dysfunction associated with chronic prostatitis
4. UPOINT, prostate massage, Botox, and shockwave treatment if available from your HMO or PPO or if available in your area on an out-network basis.

5. Referral to a pain management specialist and acupuncture for pain.

Primary care doctors
1. Initial testing and screening for STDs and UTIs.
2. Prescription for 5 mg daily Cialis.
3. Monitoring and initial testing for health conditions such as diabetes, ulcers, and irritable bowel syndrome that can impact chronic prostatitis. And referral to specialists, including pain management specialists.
4. Referral to a psychiatrist to treat depression

Specialists
1. Pain Management specialists and related acupuncture treatment.
2. Acupuncture for pain treatment
3. Psychiatrists to treat depression

Pain management, ED, depression, acupuncture for pain management, daily 5 mg Cialis, Botox, and addressing the impact of health conditions such as diabetes, ulcers, and irritable bowel syndrome in treating chronic prostatitis are all integral and important parts of the chronic Prostatitis 360 Protocol and are discussed in the chapters that follow in detail. Chapters 9 and 10 are dedicated to treating ED and depression. Conventional medical treatments are the primary treatments for these two common side effects of chronic prostatitis. You need to access these treatments through your health care providers, but this book and the Prostatitis 360 Protocol can help guide you in how to incorporate these treatments into your overall treatment program. Acupuncture may be difficult to access directly through HMO and PPO health plans. I

CHAPTER 3
Conventional Medical Treatment for Chronic Prostatitis

have listed acupuncture under pain management because I have found it's easier to obtain acupuncture services for pain by working with a pain management doctor that includes an acupuncture provider as part of their practice or has a referral or working relationship with an outside acupuncturist. If you're part of a PPO, look for pain management specialists in your network who incorporate acupuncture in their practice, or check if they refer you to an acupuncturist.

Implementing the Core Prostatitis 360 Protocol

In Part 2 of the book, the three chapters that follow are the core chronic prostatitis 360 protocol. The three-part core program consists of diet changes, supplements, and lifestyle changes. The starting point and the foundation for treating chronic prostatitis is the Prostatitis 360 Protocol anti-inflammation diet. The next chapter addresses in detail the critical importance and role of the anti-inflammation diet in treating chronic prostatitis and how to implement the diet.

PART II
The Core Protocol

CHAPTER 4
The Chronic Prostatitis 360 Protocol Diet

Diet Change is the first step in implementing the Chronic Prostatitis 360 protocol. It forms the foundation for the entire protocol. Our diet has a profound and direct impact on three key aspects of our health: inflammation, gut health, and the immune system. These, in turn, directly and indirectly influence prostate inflammation. These health issues are highly complex and not fully understood by medical science. To address them in any detail is beyond the scope of this book. Instead, we will focus in this chapter on the role of inflammation in our diet and how it impacts overall inflammation in the body, our gut health, and our immune system.

We now have over 50 years of scientific research on the impact of diet change on chronic prostatitis symptoms. While this research does not always meet the gold standard of scientific studies (double-blind placebo-controlled studies), it is still recognized as scientifically valid. It was conducted by respected doctors, urologists, and medical researchers and published in peer-reviewed medical journals. All these studies show that removing highly inflammatory foods from our diet—known as pro-inflammatory foods—and adding foods that lower inflammation can significantly reduce chronic prostatitis symptoms, including both pain and urination issues.

The largest of these studies, involving 1,710 men, was conducted by Dr. Milton Krisiloff, a urologist in Santa Monica, CA. The results of the study were published in a peer-reviewed journal in 2002. In the study, patients were required to follow a strict diet, abstaining from all alcohol, all forms of caffeine, and hot and spicy foods for 12 weeks. They were also warned that even the slightest deviation from the diet could prevent the success of the treatment. Dr. Krisiloff reported an 87% success rate, with success defined as an 80% reduction in symptoms for several different pain and urination symptoms. Dr. Krisiloff concluded that alcohol, caffeine, and hot and spicy foods cause inflammation in the prostate and urethra, leading to the common pain and urinary symptoms of chronic prostatitis. (1) An 80% reduction in symptoms for 87% of patients after three months is a success rate that has not been replicated in any study before or since. Despite this, all the studies on the use of diet change as a treatment for chronic prostatitis consistently show dramatic reductions in symptoms.

Two important earlier studies cited by Dr. Krisiloff came to similar conclusions about the role of highly inflammatory foods in causing prostate inflammation and the symptoms of chronic prostatitis. Roberts and colleagues also studied the elimination of alcoholic drinks, caffeine, and hot and spicy foods, concluding that these foods play a significant role in the symptoms of chronic prostatitis. (2) In another study by Powell and colleagues, 900 patients were treated with antihistamines and the elimination of citrus fruits, pepper, condiments, nuts, cocoa (which contains caffeine), and tomatoes. They reported that 75% of these patients experienced a significant reduction in chronic prostatitis symptoms. (3) Both Powell and Krisiloff speculated that the non-responders could be attributed to a lack of strict compliance or the possibility that some of the study patients had urethral strictures.

More recent studies conducted over the past 20 years have compared various diet and lifestyle modifications and their impact on chronic

CHAPTER 4
The Chronic Prostatitis 360 Protocol Diet

prostatitis symptoms. In these studies, alcohol is often identified as the single most important cause of symptoms of chronic prostatitis, with up to 90% of the study participants reporting significant improvement after eliminating alcoholic drinks.

I have drawn on these scientific studies, as well as insights from my personal experience with diet changes, to develop the Chronic Prostatitis 360 Diet. An anti-inflammation diet was the first treatment alternative I tried, and it was successful. In my case, I achieved a 30% reduction in symptoms after following a strict diet that removed all alcoholic drinks, all forms of caffeine (including chocolate), all types of hot and spicy foods, and several other categories of highly inflammatory foods, including acidic foods such as citrus, tomatoes, etc., added sugar, gluten, and high-histamine foods like canned fish. While I did not achieve the 87% and 75% reductions in symptoms reported by Krisiloff and Powell, a 30% reduction in symptoms was nevertheless a major breakthrough after struggling with severe chronic prostatitis for several years. After suffering for several years and not seeing any improvement from conventional medical treatments such as prostate surgery, physical therapy, commonly prescribed drugs, and antibiotics, a 30% reduction in pain was not only a major breakthrough but also a tremendous relief from my severe daily pain. For the first time in years, I had days with little or no pain.

It was at this point that I developed one of the most important insights in my experience with treating chronic prostatitis. That insight is that diet is not only important, but it may be, for many men, the foundation for all other types of treatment. An anti-inflammatory diet was not the first alternative treatment I tried. Two months before implementing the anti-inflammatory diet, I took a combination of quercetin and pollen extract (Graminex®) for 75 days with no benefit. However, after implementing the diet, when I tried quercetin again, I saw a significant improvement. When I tried pollen extract a second time a few months later, I saw a dramatic improvement in both my pain and urination symptoms. This is an example of the importance of combination therapy—what medical researchers call multimodal therapy—versus monotherapy (a single-treatment approach) in treating chronic prostatitis. Research shows that a small percentage of men, ranging from 5% to 10%, may be able to achieve a cure with just one treatment, such as diet, pollen extract, or quercetin. However, most men will need combination therapy or multimodal therapy, which combines diet, proven supplements, and lifestyle changes, to achieve an 80% to 90% reduction in symptoms or, in some cases, a complete cure.

Starting with diet, however, is a challenge since the diet component of the Prostatitis 360 Protocol is arguably the most difficult to implement. The typical American or Western diet is highly inflammatory, with alcoholic drinks, various forms of caffeine, added sugar, highly processed meats, and gluten, for example, being part of the typical daily diet. This means that the body and the prostate are, in effect, bombarded on a daily basis with high levels of inflammation. Therefore, the first step in healing the prostate and reducing inflammation is to stop this daily assault of inflammation. After 90 days of relief from daily inflammation, the prostate begins the process of healing from decades, or even a lifetime, of daily exposure to higher levels of inflammation and becomes better able to benefit from a wide range of anti-inflammatory treatments. This is the theory behind an anti-inflammatory chronic prostatitis diet. There is no direct scientific evidence to prove this theory beyond the studies that show that removing inflammatory foods results in significant improvement in symptoms. There is no scientific explanation for why some men continue to have a highly inflammatory diet for decades and never experience chronic prostatitis. For reasons that science does not fully understand, some men are sensitive to high levels of inflammation in their diet, or they may develop a sensitivity over time, while most men do not. The same phenomenon applies to benign prostatic hyperplasia (BPH), overactive bladder, and interstitial cystitis (IC) - three other common conditions that involve the bladder, prostate, and urethra.

What follows is a more detailed discussion of how a highly inflammatory diet impacts inflammation in the body, gut health, the immune system, and the impact on chronic prostatitis symptoms.

CHAPTER 4
The Chronic Prostatitis 360 Protocol Diet

Chronic Inflammation

Inflammation is a normal and necessary part of how a healthy human body functions. However, it becomes a problem when it is excessive and chronic. Chronic inflammation, including what is called low-grade chronic inflammation, is believed to cause pain directly and, over time, create greater sensitivity to pain. Excessive inflammation plays a role in a wide range of medical conditions, including hemorrhoids, irritable bowel syndrome, ulcers, acid reflux disease, and frequent diarrhea or constipation, to name just a few common examples. When reviewing individual case studies of men with chronic prostatitis, you often find that many of them suffer from many of the common inflammation-related medical conditions listed above.

In my case, I had lived with serious or borderline cases of most of these conditions. Mild hemorrhoids, diarrhea, and constipation had been lifelong, chronic problems. I found that within six months of adopting an anti-inflammation diet - adding anti-inflammatory foods that actively reduce inflammation and increase fiber - I was able to eliminate hemorrhoids, irritable bowel syndrome, ulcers, acid reflux disease, and occasional bouts of diarrhea and constipation. In my case, adopting an anti-inflammatory diet was the first and perhaps most important step in combination with several treatments that eventually led to a 90% reduction in my chronic prostatitis symptoms and, ultimately, a cure.

Every men with chronic prostatitis should have blood tests done to measure the overall inflammation in their body. The most important tests are for fibrinogen, C-reactive protein, and homocysteine. These are three of the tests I discuss and recommend for all men with chronic prostatitis in Chapter 1. You can have C-reactive protein and homocysteine levels within the normal range and still be highly susceptible to chronic inflammation in your diet affecting your body and prostate. However, high readings may indicate that this is a particularly severe issue in your case. There is a wide range of factors that impact inflammation in the body and the prostate, in addition to diet. One such factor is stress. Stress is commonly associated with conditions like ulcers, to cite just one example.

In the lifestyle chapter, we will address stress management and other lifestyle changes that can impact inflammation.

Gut Health

Our gastrointestinal system is closely linked to a wide range of important health issues, including inflammation and our immune system. An anti-inflammatory diet, by removing highly inflammatory foods and adding anti-inflammatory foods to our diet, as well as specific supplements like probiotics, can greatly improve our overall gut health, thereby reducing inflammation and improving our immune system. Many of the inflammation-related health conditions discussed above are closely linked to our gastrointestinal system. Therefore, lowering inflammation starts with a diet that removes highly inflammatory foods that damage our gut health and adding foods that lower inflammation, along with prebiotics and probiotics, to rebuild the health of our gastrointestinal system.

A high-inflammation diet can cause Irritable Bowel Syndrome (IBS), which is characterized by abdominal cramping, bloating, constipation, and diarrhea. IBS can worsen the common urination symptoms of chronic prostatitis. In this chapter, we'll discuss how to use diet to lower inflammation, including prebiotic and probiotic foods. In Chapter 5 on supplements, I will focus in greater detail on specific pre- and probiotic supplements to add to the protocol.

Immune System

The health of our immune system also impacts chronic pain conditions, such as chronic prostatitis. Our diet is one of many factors that influence our immune health. Stress management, exercise, and the quality of our sleep are other important factors that impact the health of our immune system. We will address these issues in detail in the chapter on lifestyle changes in treating chronic prostatitis. However, we know that certain aspects of our diet play an important role in boosting or lowering our immune health. It's widely believed that alcohol—especially consuming alcoholic drinks on any kind of regular basis—does a great deal to weaken our immune system. Alcohol is an insult to our bodies on all three fronts: it is highly inflammatory, it damages gastrointestinal health, and it weakens our immune system. That may be why removing alcohol from our diet could be the single most important dietary change we can make to lower our chronic prostatitis symptoms.

The Prostatitis 360 Diet: Three Core Diet Changes

Diet is the starting point and foundation for treating chronic prostatitis for most men. Much of what we eat and drink is believed to be pro-inflammatory or causing inflammation. Some of it is neutral, and some foods are actually anti-inflammatory—in other words, they fight inflammation in the body. The plan is to eliminate or dramatically reduce inflammatory foods and increase neutral and anti-inflammatory foods. The good news is that even if you eliminate all known pro-inflammatory foods and drinks from your diet, you can still have a very healthy, balanced, and satisfying diet. The bad news is that many of the things we love the most in the typical American or Western diet cause the greatest inflammation. The following are the three categories of food and drink believed to have the greatest negative impact on chronic prostatitis symptoms:

Alcohol

All alcohol, including wine and beer, is considered pro-inflammatory. While some drinks, such as red wine, champagne, and beer, are worse than others, all alcoholic drinks are highly inflammatory. You must make a commitment to completely remove alcoholic drinks for a minimum of 120 days at the start of the diet. Realistically, you should plan to abstain completely for 9 to 12 months. After 12 months, most men can have a very limited number of drinks on a few special occasions throughout the year. The plan I follow now is to have one glass of wine a day for no more than four days in a row for special occasions such as weddings, anniversaries, vacations, and holidays, with a total of four special events per year. This plan has had no negative impact on my symptoms. In social situations, ordering sparkling or flat mineral water with a slice of lemon or a wedge of lime (not squeezed) is a good alternative. Cooking with small amounts of wine that is reduced during the cooking process is fine for most men, especially after the first year.

Caffeine

This includes all forms of caffeine, including coffee, regular tea, green tea, and any other source of caffeine, such as chocolate and decaf coffees, teas, and cola soft drinks. Decaf coffee and tea still contain caffeine levels that are too high. Unlike alcoholic drinks, I believe we must come to terms with completely stopping all forms of caffeine. We have to accept and learn to enjoy alternatives, such as various caffeine-free herbal teas. Some of the best include chamomile tea, which helps with sleep and relaxation, improves digestion, and lowers inflammation, and peppermint tea, which is good for soothing the bladder. After experimenting with several different teas, I've settled on peppermint tea for its bold aromatic taste and its effectiveness in soothing my bladder, which is helpful for dealing with chronic prostatitis. If you're a chocolate lover, all forms are unfortunately off the menu—not only because of the caffeine content but also because cocoa has other potentially harmful compounds for men with chronic prostatitis. You can find sugar-free or low-sugar white chocolate online, and for some men, that is a reasonably satisfying alternative. White chocolate with nuts can actually provide some health benefits.

Hot and Spicy Foods

This includes hot and spicy condiments, seasonings, hot peppers, hot mustards, Tabasco, salsa, horseradish, chili, hot sauce, and pepperoni. In practice, this means not only removing spicy seasonings from our recipes and restaurant orders but also largely eliminating Mexican, Thai, and Indian cuisine. There's a wide range of commonly available herbs and spices to add flavor to your cooking and replace hot and spicy seasonings, including black pepper, cilantro, garlic, basil, holy basil, oregano, parsley, rosemary, and sage. All of these common spices have the added benefit of lowering inflammation. Small amounts of salt may be fine, but in general, salt should be eliminated from the diet.

CHAPTER 4
The Chronic Prostatitis 360 Protocol Diet

The Challenge of Change

Some aspects of the lifestyle changes required in the Chronic Prostatitis 360 Protocol can be difficult, but for most men, the diet changes of the protocol are the most challenging. Alcohol and caffeine are particularly difficult. These are not just important parts of the American diet; in many ways, they're important parts of our culture, how we socialize, and, for many of us, important passions in life. In my case, giving up wine and coffee meant, in some ways, fundamentally changing who I was. I was a connoisseur and collector of red wine and a lover of high-quality Italian espresso. Collecting wines from Italy and France and going on winery tours were important hobbies, travel interests, and passions of mine. I fully appreciate the challenge of giving up decades of, or in the case of men over 50, nearly a lifetime of drinking coffee and alcoholic drinks.

The question I had to ask myself was: "Is wine and coffee so important to me that I want to continue living in serious chronic pain every day for the next 30 years of my life? For the rest of my life? What does it mean for the quality of my life to live with serious daily pain?" When I framed the issue in these terms, the answer was very clear. Indeed, my answer was absolutely not! Eliminating serious daily pain from my life was much more important than wine, coffee, or any other component of my diet. Serious daily pain had a devastating impact on the quality of my life, and restoring the quality of my life was far more important.

I believe this is the question most men with chronic prostatitis must ask themselves. There is a small percentage of men with mild chronic prostatitis symptoms who may be cured with one or a combination of the five main supplements for chronic prostatitis, for example, but most men will need to make major diet and lifestyle changes. And even if your response is as clear and definitive as mine, the day-to-day challenge of giving up things like wine and coffee after decades is still very difficult and takes time and patience. In fact, while it was difficult for me initially, I was actually surprised that after six months, I found that giving up wine and coffee was manageable and increasingly easy with time.

We are faced with a series of difficult changes—changes that challenge some of our fundamental belief systems about our role, the role of the doctor, and the role of the traditional healthcare system in treating a major health problem. We must change how we think about the status of urologists as the experts in the treatment of chronic prostatitis. We must change our attitude toward doctors and traditional medical care in the treatment of serious health conditions. We have to change our attitude about our role and responsibility in treating our chronic prostatitis. We have the challenge of learning about a very different approach to healthcare. We must believe that alternative treatments for chronic prostatitis are credible and work. And perhaps the greatest challenge is the dramatic and difficult change in our diet and lifestyle. These are all difficult changes that require us to adapt to a great deal of change almost all at once.

When I think about the critical importance of adapting to change for men with chronic prostatitis, the following quote from Charles Darwin is particularly relevant and insightful:

> "It is not the strongest of the species that survive, nor the most intelligent, but the most responsive to change."

In many ways, adapting to change is at the heart of what men with chronic prostatitis must do to manage and successfully treat this condition.

The Complete Chronic Prostatitis Anti-Inflammation Diet

The diet consists of removing foods that cause inflammation and adding foods that lower inflammation. The resulting diet is a balanced one, primarily focused on whole foods, with an emphasis on fresh vegetables, fruits, and minimally processed proteins such as wild-caught fish. The diet largely eliminates packaged and processed foods. Highly inflammatory foods fall into several subcategories, including acidic, fermented, processed, spicy, preserved, and high-histamine foods. This includes all

CHAPTER 4
The Chronic Prostatitis 360 Protocol Diet

forms of added sugar, gluten or wheat, and dairy. This is a dramatic change from the typical American or Western diet. In fact, it is so different that it often raises the question: "What can you eat?" But as you will see, you can have a satisfying and balanced diet with a rich variety of foods.

We've already discussed the core of the anti-inflammatory diet, which involves eliminating alcohol, caffeine, and spicy foods. The following is a list of the other highly inflammatory foods that need to be removed from your diet. I believe that, especially during the first year, it is important to eliminate all of these foods. After the first year, you can begin to experiment with adding small amounts of categories like dairy and gluten. However, in most cases, most of these categories of inflammatory foods should be permanently removed from your diet. In each category, I will discuss alternatives, if any, and the prospect of experimenting with small amounts of food in each category after the first year.

At this point, you can choose to implement the Krisiloff diet discussed earlier by eliminating alcohol, caffeine, and spicy foods for 12 weeks. Dr. Krisiloff's research, based on over a decade of experience treating 1,700 patients, provides some validation that these three changes to your diet may be enough. However, this is an individual judgment call. If you're capable of giving up alcohol and caffeine, it is relatively easy to implement most of the full anti-inflammation diet. I made the decision to implement a complete anti-inflammatory diet once I discovered this alternative treatment for reducing my chronic prostatitis symptoms. That decision came after nearly two years of suffering with severe chronic prostatitis symptoms. I believe many men who have struggled with it for years will make the same decision. They will want to see the best possible results as quickly as possible.

We know from 50 years of scientific research that alcohol and caffeine are the worst for chronic prostatitis. However, there is no research beyond that to rank the following categories of foods by the level of inflammation they cause. The following is a list of highly inflammatory foods that should be removed and inflammation-lowering foods that should be added to this anti-inflammation diet, along with some tips and advice on managing the chronic prostatitis diet.

Citrus Fruits

This includes all varieties of lemons, limes, oranges, and grapefruit. Citrus fruits are highly acidic and inflammatory. Mild seasonings such as thyme and basil can be used as alternatives to lemon for seasoning fish. You could experiment with small amounts of lemon as a seasoning in sauces and salad dressings after the first year, but in general, citrus fruits should be removed from the diet long term.

Tomatoes

This involves not just fresh tomatoes but all tomato-based products, including pasta sauces, pizza sauce, salsa, and ketchup. All tomato-based products are highly acidic. It also includes red pizza sauce, which is the basis for making pizza. However, many restaurants now offer gluten-free dough, and you can use olive oil as a substitute for the pizza sauce. Mozzarella cheese is an acceptable form of cheese on this diet, making for a simple yet reasonably good pizza. In Italian cuisine, it's possible to substitute regular pasta with gluten-free pasta and use white sauces or olive oil instead of red tomato-based sauces.

Highly Processed Meats

This includes all cured, smoked, and canned meats and fish, such as all types of sausages and sandwich meats. Cured meats like bacon, salami, and hot dogs are highly acidic, high in histamine, and contain high levels of additives and preservatives. This category of foods should be removed from your diet long term.

Additives, Preservatives, Antibiotics, and Hormones

Additives, preservatives, antibiotics, hormones, flavor enhancers, and sodium, fructose, and other sugars are all highly inflammatory. Food additives should be avoided whenever possible. If you eat beef at all, such as once a week, it should be grass-fed beef if you can afford it. Look for chicken that has fewer or no antibiotics, and buy eggs from pasture-raised chickens.

CHAPTER 4
The Chronic Prostatitis 360 Protocol Diet

Sugar

All added sugar should be removed, as sugar is highly inflammatory. In practice, this means giving up desserts, pastries, soft drinks, candies, and a wide range of packaged foods with added sugar. Naturally occurring sugars, primarily in fruits but also in some vegetables, are fine. In fact, several fruits that are high in naturally occurring sugar, such as blueberries and watermelon, have valuable anti-inflammatory properties. High-fructose corn syrup (HFCS) is particularly inflammatory and should be strictly avoided. HFCS is used in many packaged and processed foods. It's important to avoid processed foods whenever possible and read labels carefully. Refined carbohydrates such as white bread, pasta, and white rice are quickly and easily converted to glucose in our bloodstream and should be replaced with gluten-free bread, gluten-free pasta, and brown rice. There are natural alternatives to sugar that do not raise glucose levels, including stevia, monk fruit sweetener, and allulose. However, some people find that these sweeteners cause gastrointestinal discomfort, which is an important concern on the anti-inflammation diet. They should be avoided or used in small amounts. Finally, honey remains controversial, but the consensus appears to be that pure, unrefined raw honey, used in moderation occasionally, is fine. I believe the best strategy is to approach added sugars and sweeteners like alcohol—abstaining completely during the first year—and then having a small slice of cake on birthdays and other special occasions after the first year if it has no impact on your symptoms.

Fresh Meat and Animal Proteins

Minimally processed fresh chicken, turkey, lamb, pork, and beef are acceptable. If available in your area and affordable, pasture-raised, grass-fed beef is best. Also, look for chicken and pork that are raised hormone- and antibiotic-free, or at least use fewer hormones and antibiotics. Chicken that use fewer hormones will often be labeled "natural." The ideal protein for men with chronic prostatitis is wild-caught fish. Fatty fish, ideally wild-caught, such as salmon, herring, mackerel, sardines, and tuna (not canned), are excellent sources of high-quality protein. These fatty fish are high in omega-3 fatty acids, which help lower inflammation. In fact, there is a strong case to be made that the ideal diet for men with chronic prostatitis is a vegetarian diet that includes wild-caught fatty fish as the primary animal source of protein. However, realistically, most men will want to add chicken, turkey, pork, and beef to their diet. The best compromise is a diet high in fish and poultry, with some pork and only occasional beef that is ideally grass-fed and pasture-raised.

Dairy

Most people can tolerate dairy products. However, for some, dairy can cause inflammation and gastrointestinal problems that contribute to inflammation in the bladder, prostate, and urethra. Dairy-related inflammation problems fall into the following categories: milk allergies, lactose intolerance, high saturated fat, and high histamine. Milk allergies occur when the body cannot digest certain milk proteins. If you have a milk allergy, you typically know it, and you should be aware that it also causes inflammation. If you're not sure and you're experiencing symptoms such as rashes or gastrointestinal discomfort after consuming dairy products, you should consider removing dairy from your diet. Lactose intolerance is the inability to process the lactose found in dairy products. This condition is fairly common, and most people with lactose intolerance are aware of it. If you experience bloating or gastrointestinal distress after consuming dairy products, you should consider removing dairy from your diet for 30 days to see if your symptoms improve. Full-fat dairy products are high in saturated fat, which can contribute to chronic inflammation.

The FDA recommends limiting saturated fat to 10% of your total daily calorie intake. If you have no other inflammation-related issues with dairy, it may be wise to choose fat-free or low-fat dairy options. A major concern for individuals with histamine intolerance is the high histamine content of many fermented and aged dairy products, such as cow, sheep, and goat milk-based foods. Aged hard cheeses like parmesan, gouda, Swiss, and cheddar are particularly problematic. Most fresh cheeses are tolerated on a low-histamine diet, including mozzarella, ricotta, cottage cheese, farmer's cheese, mascarpone, and plain cream cheese. All fermented dairy products, such as kefir and yogurt, are high in histamine and should be avoided on a low-histamine diet. Non-dairy milk alternatives, such as coconut, almond, rice, hemp, and oat milk, are safe and have the added advantage of containing no lactose.

In the next two sections, we will discuss in greater detail gluten—another major category of high-histamine foods—and the larger issue of histamine intolerance in general.

Gluten

Gluten is present in all foods made from wheat. It poses two problems for men with chronic prostatitis: it causes inflammation, and it's high in histamines, which cause inflammation in individuals with histamine intolerance. We will address histamines in the next section, but here, we will focus on gluten and wheat products. Wheat is one of the most common foods consumed in the Western diet and, in fact, is a component of thousands of foods produced in the US. Common wheat-based products include bread, pasta, desserts, cookies, and crackers. Celiac disease is an allergy to the gluten found in wheat. Individuals with celiac disease have an allergic reaction to consuming all forms of wheat. Many people who don't have celiac disease may still have gluten sensitivity. While it may seem daunting to give up wheat-based products, there are a wide range of alternatives available, including gluten-free bread, pasta, and crackers. Many grocery stores now offer gluten-free products in all departments, with "Gluten-Free" prominently highlighted on the front of the package.

Histamine

Histamine intolerance is not widespread in the US, affecting approximately 3 to 6% of the population. Histamine intolerance occurs when the body cannot break down histamine, leading to symptoms such as headaches, intestinal discomfort, inflammation, and sinus swelling. It can contribute to inflammation in the body, particularly in the intestinal tract, bladder, and prostate.

Histamine intolerance is caused by a lack of an enzyme in the intestinal tract called DAO, which breaks down histamine. Therefore, foods that are high in histamine, as well as foods that block normal DAO function, are problematic. DAO is available as a supplement to help break down histamine. While histamine intolerance is not very common, some levels of histamine sensitivity may be more widespread. In addition to swelling in the intestinal tract, bladder, and urethra, research has identified a direct link between histamine and prostatitis. This research is ongoing.

A related condition is MAST Cell Activation Syndrome (MCAS). MAST cells are part of the immune system and release histamine and other chemicals in response to allergens. MCAS occurs when mast cells become overactive and are easily triggered by things other than normal allergens, leading to allergic-like reactions that cause swelling and inflammation of the skin, intestinal tract, and bladder. MAST cells are found throughout the body, with large concentrations in the intestinal tract and bladder. MCAS is believed to have a direct potential link to the pain and urination symptoms of prostatitis caused by MCAS-related bladder and urethra inflammation. It is important to note that alcohol and spicy foods are believed to be major triggers for MCAS. Both histamine intolerance and MCAS are complex conditions that are not fully understood. In this book, we will focus on how these two conditions may impact chronic prostatitis symptoms and offer practical steps to manage your diet to avoid the pain and urination symptoms of chronic prostatitis.

In addition to removing gluten for histamine intolerance and alcohol and spicy foods for MCAS, several other foods are high in histamine. Many of these foods are already restricted in the anti-inflammatory diet. Below is a list of the most common high-histamine foods:

CHAPTER 4
The Chronic Prostatitis 360 Protocol Diet

Foods high in histamine include:
- Alcohol and other fermented beverages
- Fermented foods and dairy products, such as yogurt and sauerkraut
- Dried fruits
- Avocados
- Eggplant
- Spinach
- Processed or smoked meats, including all sausages, sandwich meats, and bacon
- Shellfish
- Aged cheese

Foods that trigger histamine release in the body include:
- Alcohol
- Hot peppers and spicy foods
- Bananas
- Tomatoes
- Wheat germ
- Beans
- Papaya
- Chocolate
- Citrus fruits
- Nuts, specifically walnuts, cashews, and peanuts
- Food dyes and other additives

Foods that block DAO production include:
- Alcohol
- Black tea
- Mate tea
- Green tea
- Energy drinks

If, after implementing the anti-inflammation diet, you continue to experience symptoms such as headaches, bladder and intestinal bloating, and sinus swelling, you should work with your primary care doctor and specialists to perform additional testing to determine if you have histamine intolerance or MCAS. If you experience bladder issues such as bloating and pain, as discussed in Chapter 1, you should also be evaluated for the possibility of having interstitial cystitis (IC). If you are not diagnosed with overactive bladder, IC, histamine intolerance, or MCAS, your bladder may still be sensitive to certain foods. I have attached in appendix II a list of bladder-irritating foods and drinks. You may find that removing one or some of these bladder-irritating foods will improve the health of your bladder and help with some of your pain and urination symptoms. In my case, for example, red grapes increase the frequency of urination overnight and during the day, but I can have white grapes daily without any problems.

Anti-inflammation Foods

In the first part of the chronic Prostatitis 360 Diet, we focused on highly inflammatory foods that'd have to be removed from our diet. In this section, we focus on foods that are neutral or actually lower inflammation in our bodies. The following is a list of the top 10 anti-inflammation foods:

Top 10 Anti-inflammation Foods

1. **Leafy greens:** romaine, arugula, spinach and kale. If you have histamine intolerance, You may need to be careful with spinach because it is high in histamine.
2. **Extra virgin olive oil.** EVOO Should be your primary oil for salads and most cooking. Organic first cold-pressed olive oil is best.
3. **Foods containing vitamin C:** All berries (except strawberries), kiwi, broccoli, and mild bell peppers. Blueberries have the strongest anti-inflammation properties and should be a regular part of your daily diet. Vitamin C from foods is fine, but vitamin

CHAPTER 4
The Chronic Prostatitis 360 Protocol Diet

C supplements should, in general, be avoided because they can irritate the stomach and the bladder.
4. **Cruciferous vegetables:** cauliflower, broccoli, and brussels sprouts.
5. **Fatty fish:** salmon, herring, sardines, anchovies, and tuna. Fresh rather than canned. Wild-caught rather than farm-raised whenever available and if you can afford it.
6. **Prebiotic foods:** mushrooms, artichokes, onions (cooked), asparagus, apples, watermelon, chickpeas, oats, garlic, leeks, and flax seeds.
7. **Probiotic foods:** Yogurt, kefir, sauerkraut, pickles, and most other fermented foods. For those with dairy allergies, sauerkraut and pickles are good options. For those with histamine intolerance, all fermented foods are high in histamine, and probiotic supplements may be the best option. In fact, even if you regularly consume probiotic foods, probiotic supplements are still part of the Prostatitis 360 Protocol.
8. **Nuts and seeds:** most nuts and seeds are fine except peanuts. Pine nuts, pistachios(unsalted), pumpkin, and flax seeds are the best nuts and seeds. Almonds can be highly acidic and should be consumed blanched (skin removed). Unsalted pistachios are high in Zinc, an important trace mineral in prostate health.
9. **Vitamin A-rich foods:** sweet potato, carrots, and butter squash.
10. **Zinc-rich foods:** lentils, oatmeal, fresh oysters, chickpeas, pistachios, pumpkin and hemp seeds, and eggs. Zinc is a particularly important trace mineral for men with chronic prostatitis, which we'll discuss in detail in the chapter on supplements.

Anti-inflammation Superfoods

12 Superfoods
Kale, blueberries, broccoli, wild-caught salmon, pumpkin seeds, flax seeds, oatmeal, sauerkraut (If not sensitive to histamines), extra virgin olive oil, watermelon, and cooked shallots. If kale is not readily available in your area, romaine and arugula are good alternatives. You should have most of these superfoods daily, with salmon two to three times a week and sauerkraut four times a week.

Green Tea
Green tea is often included as an anti-inflammatory food, but the caffeine content makes it unacceptable on the chronic prostatitis anti-inflammation diet. Decaf green tea may be an option, but as discussed earlier, decaf teas still have significant amounts of caffeine. Given the anti-inflammation and many other health benefits of green tea, you may want to try decaf green tea after the first year to determine if you can tolerate the caffeine content. Another option is EEGG, which is a supplement derived from green tea and provides benefits without caffeine.

Quercetin
Quercetin deserves special consideration as an important part of an anti-inflammation diet. Among the five core supplements for chronic prostatitis, quercetin is the only one available from a variety of food sources. Onions and dark berries such as blueberries and blackberries are rich sources of quercetin. Other good sources include dark leafy greens, red grapes, olive oil, parsley, and sage. Dietary sources of Quercetin won't replace the high daily dose needed to treat chronic prostatitis, but adding some quercetin from our diet will complement the overall treatment protocol.

CHAPTER 4
The Chronic Prostatitis 360 Protocol Diet

Fiber

Fiber is particularly important in the anti-inflammation diet. Most men do not eat enough fiber-rich foods. A high-fiber diet has important anti-inflammation benefits, and it's critical to a healthy intestinal tract. The natural treatment of most common intestinal health problems (hemorrhoids, IBS, etc.) starts with gradually adding a substantial amount of high-quality daily fiber from several different food sources. Several daily servings of fresh whole fruits and vegetables are an important place to start. Three fiber superfoods should be incorporated into your daily diet: Organic oatmeal, ground flax seeds, and organic whole psyllium husk. It's important to buy only 100% whole psyllium husk and avoid several different commercial brands of psyllium that are often sold as laxatives. Most of these products contain additives, artificial colors, and sugars. You can find ground flaxseed and psyllium husk online in health food stores and grocery store chains such as Sprouts. One heaping tablespoon of ground flaxseed and psyllium husk is normally all you need combined with oatmeal in smoothies and on top of salads.

The Mediterranean Diet

The classic Mediterranean diet is a largely plant-based diet combined with a great deal of olive oil. It is based on research done in the 1950s on the island of Crete in Greece. I the 1950's Cretan diet was a local seasonal diet that primarily consisting of organic fruits and vegetables. Protein came from vegetables, local wild-caught fish such as anchovies, and small amounts of pasture-raised eggs and chicken. Nuts, seeds, and beans were staples of the diet. Red wine, in moderation, was also consumed daily. All 10 of the top anti-inflammatory foods, except red wine, discussed above were important parts of the Cretan diet, making it an ideal anti-inflammatory diet. Studies done in the 1950s involving men on the island of Crete between 40 and 59 reported dramatically lower incidences of heart disease than in any country studied in the Mediterranean, Europe, and the US. In the 1950s, it was not unusual for 100-year-old male farmers to still work in the fields daily. Extensive research done since the 1950s on Mediterranean diets largely based on the Cretan diet model has consistently shown that this traditional Mediterranean diet is one of the healthiest diets in the world. The Chronic Prostatitis 360 Protocol Diet is based on this Mediterranean diet with some important modifications, such as removing alcohol, caffeine, and citrus.

The Chronic Prostatitis 360 Protocol Diet Cookbook

I'm in the process of writing a cookbook to help men prepare traditional Mediterranean diet meals with the changes, modifications, and alternatives necessary for the chronic prostatitis anti-inflammatory diet. The cookbook will guide men with chronic prostatitis in preparing a wide variety of delicious low-inflammation meals based on the limitations of the chronic prostatitis diet. The cookbook will be available shortly after the release of this book.

Managing the Chronic Prostatitis Diet: Guidelines, Suggestions and Tips

General Guidelines

Prepare most of your meals at home. Make your lunch at home and take it to work. Cook from scratch. Use whole food ingredients, and 80 to 90% of your meals are made from whole food ingredients. Ask your spouse and family to incorporate some healthy foods into family meals. An anti-inflammation diet is an excellent diet for everyone, not just individuals with chronic inflammation issues. Ask your spouse and family to help and support you in keeping on track with this difficult diet and lifestyle change. Read the food ingredient list carefully to identify unwanted wheat, sugars, dairy, additives, and preservatives. Shop at grocery store chains such as Sprouts, Whole Foods, and Trader Joe's for a wider selection of organic, whole, and natural foods, as well as grass-fed beef, chicken with little or no antibiotics, and eggs from pasture-raised chickens. Trader Joe's has frozen wild-caught salmon, tuna, and halibut, among others, at relatively reasonable prices. You can find grass-fed steak and add sprouts again at

CHAPTER 4
The Chronic Prostatitis 360 Protocol Diet

relatively reasonable prices. Trader Joe's also has low or no-antibiotic chicken labeled "natural" at prices that are not much more than conventional chicken.

Restaurants

Your dining options will be limited at most restaurants. Plan ahead carefully by looking at the menu online in advance and confirming the menu items suitable for an anti-inflammation diet are available. Two good options are salmon and steak. These are normally prepared without any sauces or spices on top, and if they are, you can request to have them removed or put on the side. Salmon is an anti-inflammation superfood that is an ideal choice for restaurant dining. Steak is usually prepared plain and is sometimes available grass-fed. Vegetable sides such as broccoli and asparagus, which are common in restaurants, are also excellent choices. Most salads, of course, are fine as long as you ask for no salad dressing and ask for olive oil on the side as your salad dressing. Italian restaurants can be a challenge, but most offer steak and occasionally salmon. Most pizza restaurants now offer gluten-free crust, which, combined with olive oil as the sauce or made with a white sauce, mozzarella, and fresh basil, makes for a reasonably good Margarita pizza without gluten or red tomato sauce. Many restaurants now offer clearly marked gluten-free and vegetarian options. Ordering a bottle of mineral water is a good alternative to ordering beer or wine.

Substitutes and Alternatives

Replace pasta with gluten-free pasta. Sprouts carries a brand of Italian organic brown rice pasta, while Trader Joe's has pre-cooked, organic brown rice prepackaged in servings for two. Extra virgin olive oil is an anti-inflammation diet superfood that is an excellent alternative to salad dressings and tomato-based pasta sauces. You can also sprinkle EVOO on steamed broccoli, cauliflower, and asparagus to add flavor to these side dishes. Steaming rather than sautéing and broiling is healthier on an anti-inflammation diet. Herbs are excellent alternatives to spicy seasonings that add aroma and flavor to your dishes. Ghee, preferably from grass-fed cows, is a good alternative to butter and margarine. Most large grocery stores also have plant-based alternatives to butter and margarine. EVOO is an ideal oil for most uses, and coconut oil is a good option for high-heat cooking.

Breakfast

While most traditional American breakfast foods are off the menu, including bacon, breakfast sausage, syrup, and, of course, coffee, among others, there are some very good breakfast options. An omelet with onions sauteed in olive oil is a good choice. You can add mozzarella cheese or a small amount of feta cheese for the flavor. Served with a side of lightly toasted gluten-free bread. Thyme and basil complement omelets well and are good alternatives to salt and pepper. French toast made with gluten-free bread and lightly sauteed in olive oil is normally moist enough to eat without butter or syrup. You can also top it with ghee as an alternative to butter and syrup. Pancakes and waffles can be made with gluten-free flour cooked in olive oil and topped with ghee. The breakfast superfood for the anti-inflammation diet is oatmeal, typically 4 tablespoons combined with one tablespoon each of ground flaxseed and psyllium husk. Mix, add boiling water, and top with blueberries. Let the mixture cool until it's no longer hot. The mixture absorbs a great deal of water; you will have to experiment with the right amount of water for the consistency you like. This breakfast is an anti-inflammation powerhouse that includes a long list of important benefits, including a great deal of fiber, Omega-3 fatty acids, and zinc, to name just some of the most important benefits. Finally, fruits such as berries, grapes, and watermelon are excellent additions to breakfast.

Lunch

Gluten-free pasta with olive oil dressing and topped with basil and pine nuts and a side of lightly toasted gluten-free bread is an excellent option for lunch. It can also be prepared in advance and taken to work. A salad with a little crumbled feta cheese and olive oil dressing, aside from

CHAPTER 4
The Chronic Prostatitis 360 Protocol Diet

vegetables, such as broccoli, cauliflower, or asparagus, should be a part of your daily lunch. They can also be prepared in advance and taken to work. A serving of fruit should also be a regular part of lunch. Pre-cooked organic brown rice is pre-packaged for individual servings and microwaved, and it's a great easy lunch option that you can buy at Trader Joe's. Organic brown rice can be combined with a small serving of chicken or fish for another great lunch option. It's easy to prepare several servings of chicken thighs or chicken breast to take to work along with the organic brown rice.

Dinner

Dinner should always include a large salad, a large side of vegetables, and fruit. Skinless chicken breast and tights are great options for dinner, baked or sauteed with olive oil. Fish can be lightly sauteed on the stovetop or baked in an airtight foil pouch with olive oil and seasonings such as oregano, thyme, basil, or Herb de Provence. Occasional lean pork and grass-fed beef can be added for a variety, as well as having one or two vegetarian main courses per week.

Barbeque

The charring and burning of beef, chicken, and vegetables on a BBQ is acidic and inflammatory and produces unhealthy carcinogens. The alternative is to cook meat and vegetables in foil, including airtight foil pouches for meat and fish to seal in juices and prevent meat from drying out. This form of barbecuing preserves the experience of cooking outdoors, has some of the same barbecue aroma, and tastes great. It's not the same barbeque taste, but it still has a great taste.

Anti-inflammation Diet Results

For most men, it will take months to see the benefits of the diet. Typically, it will take a minimum of 90 to 120 days to begin to see results, and it may take up to six months to see significant improvement in your symptoms. If you have a typical American diet, especially alcohol, caffeine, spicy and acidic foods, your body has been bombarded by daily dietary inflammation for decades, and recovering from that constant assault will take time. I began to see some signs of improvement in my symptoms after six weeks, but in my case, I had already stopped drinking caffeine and significantly reduced wine. I achieved a 30% reduction in the severity of my symptoms after 90 days, and the improvement essentially plateaued at that level until I started taking 500 mg of quercetin twice a day three months later. Prior to implementing the anti-inflammation diet, I tried Quercetin for 75 days at the same dosage with no benefit, and after implementing the diet, I began to see improvement in my symptoms within 30 days.

Whether you see significant or only mild improvement, I believe that the anti-inflammation diet is the foundation on which to build the Prostatitis 360 Protocol for most men. The next phase of the protocol is the use of supplements to treat chronic prostatitis. In Chapter 5, we address the role and implementation of the supplement treatment protocol.

Chapter 5
Supplements for Chronic Prostatitis

In this chapter, we discuss the use of supplements to treat chronic prostatitis as part of the Prostatitis 360 Protocol. The medical or scientific term for supplements that have been studied or proven to treat a medical condition is *nutraceuticals*. *Phytotherapy* refers to nutraceuticals derived from plants. The five core, tier 1 nutraceutical therapies for chronic prostatitis are all phytotherapies. While diet is the necessary starting point or foundation for treating chronic prostatitis for most men, phytotherapy in the form of the five core nutraceuticals is the most beneficial part of the treatment protocol.

If you have been struggling with severe chronic prostatitis symptoms for a long time, it may be tempting to simply gather the dosage information and specific recommended brands of these five phytotherapies in this chapter and begin taking them rather than reading the entire chapter. However, I urge your to the entire chapter. In reviewing the research on these five supplements, as well as the tier 2 (add-on) supplements, I provide important insights into how they work and what to do if they don't work in your case. These insights may make the difference between success and failure with the supplement part of the protocol.

The supplements are divided into two groups. The first group consists of the five scientifically proven tier 1 or core supplements for treating chronic prostatitis. These are nettle root extract, pumpkin seed oil, pollen extract, quercetin, and the LSESR form of saw palmetto, which is a special formulation of saw palmetto. For men with chronic prostatitis, there is a strong likelihood that one, or in most cases, a combination of these five supplements will significantly improve their symptoms. The remaining supplements, or tier 2, consist of supplements that have been scientifically studied for chronic prostatitis and have demonstrated some, but limited, benefits. These include supplements that are believed to lower inflammation in general, as well as specifically in the intestinal tract and bladder. The tier 2 supplements also include those that enhance the absorption of other supplements or make the five core tier 1 supplements more effective when taken together.

There are five core phytotherapy supplements that have been proven in extensive scientific research over the past three decades to be the most effective treatments for chronic prostatitis in most men, with up to 94% of the men studied reporting an improvement of at least 25%. In most of these studies, the majority of the men reported at least a 67% improvement. Many of the studies on these supplements are randomized controlled trials (RCTs), which are the most rigorous type of scientific research for treatments of medical conditions and are considered the gold standard of scientific research. The following is a review and analysis of the research results for each of these five supplements. I have also included, where available, a review of the research results that compare these supplements with the conventional pharmaceuticals prescribed by

Chapter 5
Supplements for Chronic Prostatitis

most urologists. While there is very little research that directly compares the effectiveness of these five supplements, I have included those studies where available. In terms of the extent of the research done and the level of effectiveness, studies show that flower pollen and saw palmetto are more effective than quercetin, nettle root extract (NRE), and pumpkin seed oil (PSO).

I believe there is enough rigorous scientific research to draw the conclusion that most men will benefit from one, and in most cases a combination of, these supplements. Each of these five supplements addresses inflammation in similar and different ways. For reasons that we do not fully understand - and that science does not yet understand - what may work for one man may not work for another. The supplement that provides a great deal of improvement for one man may only offer minimal improvement for another. In my case, flower pollen extract and LSESR saw palmetto have both been very effective and much more effective than PSO and NRE, while quercetin provided only a small benefit. More extensive, rigorous research has been done on pollen extract and saw palmetto, and studies have shown that they are more effective than NRE, PSO, and quercetin. Therefore, I start with these two supplements as part of the five core tier 1 supplements.

The Core Tier 1 Supplements

Pollen Extract

Flower pollen has been used in Europe for over 40 years to treat chronic prostatitis. It has been studied for treating chronic prostatitis in Europe since the 1980s. It is manufactured by pharmaceutical companies in several countries including Sweden and Germany. In Europe, it is classified as a drug and is widely prescribed by urologists throughout the continent. The most widely studied and used pollen extract in Europe and Asia is Cernilton, made by AB

Cernelle in Sweden. Most of the flower pollen extract sold in the U.S. is produced by Graminex LLC, which sells it under the brand name *PollenAid* or licenses it to other supplement companies under the name *Graminex G63*. There has been extensive research in the U.S. and Europe over the past 15 years using Graminex G63. Research results have been similar for both supplements.

Scientific Research

There have been over 30 scientific studies on flower pollen as a treatment for chronic prostatitis since the 1980s. These studies were published in peer-reviewed scientific journals and conducted by highly respected medical researchers, primarily in Europe, North America, and Japan. A review and analysis of several individual studies, as well as meta-analyses (analysis of multiple studies), show that flower pollen is highly effective in treating chronic prostatitis, with an average of 79% of the patients studied experiencing an improvement of at least 25%. The success rate across multiple studies is also fairly consistent. A meta-analysis of 15 studies conducted in 2017 showed that the range of improvement was between 62% and 96%. These ranges were similar for both RCT studies (highly rigorous scientific studies) and other non-RCT scientific studies. The average improvement was 74% in RCT studies and 83% in non-RCT studies. (1)

A Possible Cure for Chronic Prostatitis for Some Men

Most of the studies on flower pollen have been short, typically lasting 12 weeks. These short-term studies have reported significant improvement in a large percentage of the patients, but none of these short-term studies have reported dramatic improvement or a cure. However, there are several long-term studies that provide

Chapter 5
Supplements for Chronic Prostatitis

compelling evidence that flower pollen, even as a monotherapy, can provide a cure for a significant percentage of men -ranging from 20% to 46% - who take it for six months or more.

These long-term studies are important because they evaluate potential long-term side effects and improvements in symptoms. In my case, it took three months to see significant benefits from flower pollen and six months to see the full benefit. The typical 12-week study cannot always accurately measure the effectiveness of flower pollen. One key study is an 18-month non-RCT study conducted in 1989 by Buck and colleagues, which involved 15 patients who took two tablets of Cernilton (1,000 mg) twice a day for 18 months. After 18 months, 46% were symptom-free, 40% had significant improvement, and 13% showed no improvement. Most patients who benefited saw significant improvement after three months. **(2)**

Another important study, conducted in 2006 by Elist and colleagues, was a six-month RCT with 60 patients. All patients had chronic prostatitis for at least six months, ranging from six months to 5.5 years. The patients took 74mg of *Prostat/Prolit* (a pollen extract with ingredients similar to Cernilton) three times a day. The symptom evaluation was thorough, covering seven pain locations, six voiding symptoms, three storage symptoms, and four sex-related symptoms. After six months, 20% of patients were cured, 74% reported significant improvement, and 26% had no improvement. In the placebo group, 64% had no improvement, 36% reported significant improvement, and none were cured. Notably, in the case of the cured patients, a cure was defined not only by improvements in pain and urination symptoms but also by improvements in sexual symptoms. **(3)** It's important to note that in this study, the dosage was only 222 mg, compared to the 1,000 mg used in the Buck study, and the Buck study lasted three times longer (18 months compared to six months). These two factors alone may explain the differences in outcomes between the two studies.

In another important study, conducted by Rugendorf and colleagues in 1993, 90 patients who were given 500 mg of Cernilton three times a day (a total of 1,500 mg) for six months. The study included patients with complicating factors such as bladder neck sclerosis, prostatic calculi, or urethral strictures. After six months, 42% of patients reported significant improvement, 36% were cured, and 22% saw no improvement. Only 6% of patients with complicating factors had a positive response. (4) These studies provide significant evidence that between 20% and 46% of men can achieve a cure with flower pollen as a stand-alone or monotherapy if taken for six months or more.

In my case, when I first took flower pollen alone as a monotherapy, it did not provide a cure or even a significant benefit. I was in the category of men in these studies who failed to see any improvement. But once I combined a non-inflammatory diet with flower pollen, I saw dramatic, life-changing improvement in my symptoms. Flower pollen proved to be the single most important component of my successful treatment protocol. Therefore, I believe that adding the other elements of the Prostatitis 360 Protocol—starting with diet—can provide dramatic symptom improvement for many men and possibly a cure for some men.

It's also important to note that these three studies do not provide any information on the response rate by symptom severity. It's possible that the men who achieved a cure had moderate or less severe symptoms. In my case, my symptoms were severe, which may explain why I failed to respond to flower pollen as a stand-alone treatment. I had to combine diet change, lifestyle changes, flower

Chapter 5
Supplements for Chronic Prostatitis

pollen, saw palmetto, pumpkin seed oil, and nettle root extract to achieve a cure.

Complicating Factors

The Rugendorf study is particularly important because it took into account complicating factors when measuring the effectiveness of flower pollen. There are three complicating factors—bladder neck sclerosis, prostatic calculi, and urethral strictures—that can cause the symptoms of chronic prostatitis or be major contributing factors. These conditions should be included in the battery of tests for chronic prostatitis, though insurance companies often do not pay for these tests, and they are rarely performed. It is widely believed that these three conditions are rare, but there are no large-scale rigorous population studies to verify whether they are more common than believed. Because we don't have large-scale, rigorous research with credible data about how common these conditions are, it's possible that these complicating factors are more common than widely believed. I discuss the three complicating factors in greater detail in Chapter 1.

Urethral strictures are believed to affect approximately 1% of the male population and are twice as likely among men over 65. However, the true prevalence of this condition is poorly understood. Urethral strictures involve both pain and urination symptoms. Prostatic calculi (stones found in the prostate gland) are believed to be quite common, with estimates suggesting that 7% to 82% of men have them. However, most men with prostatic calculi don't experience symptoms, and the presence of the calculi is often discovered when testing for benign prostatic hyperplasia (BPH). A prostate ultrasound can detect these stones. The primary symptoms are urinary, but pain can also occur. Bladder neck strictures (BNOS) are a physical blockage at the start of the urethra and just above the prostate. It is believed to affect 3.9% to 7.6% of men, with the primary symptoms being urination-related.

In the Rugendorf study, 24% of the men tested had complicating factors. There were 90 patients in the study, so in strict scientific terms, the sample size is too small to extrapolate that 24% of the male population has these complicating factors. However, this is an interesting data point about how widespread these complicating factors may be. In the study, only 6% of men with complicating factors showed improvement. If you don't see significant improvement in your symptoms after implementing the anti-inflammatory diet and taking all or most of the core tier 1 supplements for six months, I recommend going back and being tested for these complicating factors. In fact, Rugendorf and colleagues recommended that if you don't see improvement after just three months with flower pollen alone, you should be tested for these complicating factors. If you're among the 92% of men with PPO or HMO healthcare, it's likely that your request for urethral strictures and BPNO tests will be denied. I recommend appealing, and if it's denied again, you can pay for the tests out of pocket if you can afford them. If you do appeal, I suggest using the data from the Rugendorf study as part of your appeal. **(5)** The Rugendorf study was published in the highly respected *British Journal of Urology*. The authors, Rugendorf and Buck, are two of the most respected researchers in the field of chronic prostatitis. The test for prostatic calculi or prostate stones involves a simple, inexpensive prostate ultrasound that is normally covered by insurance.

Unfortunately, the scientific studies of saw palmetto, PSO, NRE, and quercetin do not analyze men with complicating factors. It's possible that if the other supplements were tested for complicating

Chapter 5
Supplements for Chronic Prostatitis

factors, they would show similar results. However, we need scientific studies to validate that assumption.

There is substantial scientific evidence that flower pollen extract, including Graminex and Cernilton, is the most effective phytotherapy for chronic prostatitis when compared to saw palmetto extract, PSO, NRE, and quercetin. It is the only one proven in 6- to 18-month studies to provide a cure for 20% to 46% of men. It is the single most effective supplement for treating chronic prostatitis. I believe that flower pollen extract, combined with the Prostatitis 360 Diet, will be the foundation on which most men can build the Prostatitis 360 Protocol for treating their chronic prostatitis. The key is to combine flower pollen with the Prostatitis 360 Diet and allow six months to see the full benefit of this combination. Studies show that most men will begin to see improvement after three months.

Dosage and Brands

The only flower pollen extract in the U.S. that has been extensively studied and proven effective is made by Graminex, LLC. The company sells its flower pollen extract under the brand name *PollenAid* with a dosage of 500 mg. The active ingredient in *PollenAid* is Graminex G63. The company also sells Graminex G63 to other supplement makers. In my case, I use *PollenAid* and take 500 mg each with breakfast, lunch, and dinner for a total of 1,500 mg. Most studies, including those cited above, that reported the greatest effectiveness used either 1,000 or 1,500 mg. You can start with 1,000 mg and experiment with 1,500 mg to see if you have better results.

Combination Treatments

Pollen Extract & Hyaluronic Acid and B Vitamins

A 2019 study in Europe compared flower pollen (1,000 mg) combined with B vitamins (B1, B6, B12) and hyaluronic acid to bromelain, a supplement derived from pineapples believed to have anti-inflammatory properties. In the flower pollen group, 75% of patients experienced at least a 25% improvement, compared to 24% in the bromelain group. It's unclear if adding the B vitamin combination and hyaluronic acid significantly improves outcomes over pollen extract alone. Several RCT studies of pollen alone have shown comparable or better results. A study comparing pollen alone with the combination of pollen extract, hyaluronic acid, and B vitamins would be more useful in determining any potential benefit from adding these components. (5) If you find that flower pollen is effective in your case, you can experiment with adding B vitamins and hyaluronic acid to see if they enhance its effectiveness.

Saw Palmetto Extract

Saw Palmetto extract has been used to treat chronic prostatitis and BPH in Europe for over 35 years. In Europe and parts of Asia, LSESr saw Palmetto extract has the status of a prescription drug. It is manufactured by pharmaceutical companies, rather than supplement makers, in Germany, France, Italy, Spain, and Japan. The European Medicines Agency, the European equivalent of the FDA, has approved LSESr Saw Palmetto extract as the equivalent of prescription drug. The European Urology Association, the European equivalent of the American Urology Association, has officially recommended LSESr Saw Palmetto extract for BPH and LUTS, which is a broad category that includes chronic prostatitis. While it's available over the counter, it is commonly prescribed by urologists throughout Europe. In Germany, for example, 50% of urologists prescribe it for BPH and chronic prostatitis. The

Chapter 5
Supplements for Chronic Prostatitis

LipidoSterolic Extract of Serenoa repens (LSESr) berries of the saw palmetto plant with a minimum of 85% fatty acids is the only scientifically proven saw palmetto extract to treat chronic prostatitis, LUTS, and BPH. There are several saw palmetto products in Europe, including Permixon, Eviprostat, and Profluss, that meet the LSESr 85% scientific standard. In the US, there is one saw palmetto extract product, Flowmentum ®, that is USP verified and has been proven in independent testing to meet the LSESr 85% fatty acid standard. A study by Chughtai and colleagues done in 2023 compared 28 randomly selected widely available brands of saw palmetto that were analyzed by an independent lab. The study found that 27 of the 28 saw palmetto brands failed to meet the 85% fatty acids standard, and only Flowmentum ® met the standard. (6)

Scientific Research

There has been an extensive body of chronic prostatitis research on saw palmetto since the 1990s. A 2015 RCT study done by Iwamura and colleagues compared LSESr saw palmetto (Eviprostat) 2x 320mg per day to flower pollen extract (Cernilton) 2x 360mg per day of pollen extract in 100 male chronic prostatitis patients divided into two groups of 50 each. After eight weeks, the Saw Palmetto group reported that 88.2% saw a 25% or greater improvement compared to 78.1% for the flower pollen group. There were no significant differences in the pain, urinary, or quality of life scores. The researchers concluded that overall, saw palmetto and flower pollen were equally effective. However, the results for the Saw Palmetto group were a little better because, on average, the CPSI scores at the start of the study were approximately 20% higher in the flower pollen group. (7)

In a RCT study by Reissigl and colleagues in 2004, 61 chronic prostatitis patients taking 320mg of saw palmetto (Permixon) for 6 months reported significant benefits. The researchers reported that 75% of the Permixon group showed at least a mild improvement, and 55% showed a substantial improvement in their CPSI scores compared to 20% and 16% for the placebo group, respectively. (8) It's important to note that while the Iwamura study reported comparable results in an 8-week study comparing saw palmetto and flower pollen, long-term studies provide evidence that flower pollen can provide a cure for 20% to 46% of men, which is vastly superior compared to saw palmetto. The six-month Reissigil study is one of the few long-term studies, and it did not result in any of the men reporting a cure. A 12-week study of 221 patients with chronic prostatitis done by Zhang et al. in 2021 showed that 73% of the patients had improvements of 25% or more in their symptoms. This was a double-blind, randomized, placebo-controlled, multicenter, clinical phase 4 study, which is the gold standard in scientific medical studies. Patients in this study with moderate symptoms began to report improvement at two weeks, and those with severe symptoms after 4 weeks. (9)

A Study of the Multimodal Treatment Model

There are very few studies of treatments for men with chronic prostatitis that combine supplements with diet and lifestyle changes. There is one study that comes close to providing scientific evidence for the effectiveness of a treatment program that is more limited but similar to the Prostatitis 360 Protocol. An Italian study done by Lambertini and colleagues in 2023 involved 245 patients diagnosed with moderate to severe chronic prostatitis. In the study, the patients were asked to make specific diet and lifestyle changes and take a combination of supplements for three months. The patients were

Chapter 5
Supplements for Chronic Prostatitis

asked to stop spicy foods, alcohol, caffeine, and cycling and take a supplement combination that consisted of 400 mg of Saw Palmetto extract with 92% fatty acids, lycopene 10mg, and bromelain 200mg. After three months, the researchers reported that the chronic prostatitis CPSI scores declined from an average of 20.3 to 13.2, the IPSS scores, used to measure urinary symptoms, declined from 19.5 to 14.3, and quality of life scores declined from 3.8 to 2.6. (10) These are significant improvements in pain, urination, and quality of life scores, especially for a relatively short 3-month study. This study is important because, to my knowledge, it's the first study that combines supplements with diet and lifestyle changes that are comparable to the Prostatitis 360 Protocol treatment model for chronic prostatitis. The study has several important limitations, such as not using a placebo group, but the most important drawback to the study is that it was too short to accurately measure the effect of a diet change and a combination of supplements that included saw palmetto. I believe it takes a minimum of 3 months just to begin to see some limited benefit from a diet change. Nevertheless, the study found substantial improvements in pain, urinary, and quality of life scores. In my case, I just began to see very small improvements three months after changing my diet to an anti-inflammation diet. It also took a full three months before I began to see significant benefits when I started to take saw palmetto. I believe you need a minimum of six months to accurately measure the impact of a supplement, lifestyle, and diet change treatment protocol for chronic prostatitis. The fact that this study found significant improvement in just three months makes a strong case for combining diet changes with supplements to treat chronic prostatitis.

In terms of the number of studies done, the quality of those studies, and the level of success reported in those studies, flower pollen extract is significantly superior compared to saw palmetto extract in terms of improving the symptoms of chronic prostatitis. While saw palmetto extract is not as effective as flower pollen extract in treating the pain and urination symptoms of chronic prostatitis, studies show that it does help with both pain and urination symptoms. If the five core phytotherapies worked in exactly the same ways, they would duplicate each other, and there would be no need to use all of them. All five achieve similar results to varying degrees, but all five are very different in how they work. Each one helps with urination and pain symptoms in different ways, and when added together, they can theoretically maximize the reduction in pain and urination symptoms. The other key rationale for using all five phytotherapy is that different men would respond in different ways to the five phytotherapy because each one works in different ways. In addition to working in a different way to improve pain and urination symptoms, saw palmetto extract may be particularly important for treating urination symptoms of chronic prostatitis. It has been extensively studied and proven to be very successful in improving the urination symptoms of BPH. There is a great deal of overlap in the urination symptoms, BPH, and chronic prostatitis, and the pharmaceuticals and supplements used to treat the two conditions. Several of the supplements used to treat BPH are also effective in treating chronic prostatitis and vice versa. The theory is that given how successful saw palmetto is in treating the urination symptoms of BPH. It may play a particularly important role among the top three phytotherapy in improving the urination symptoms of chronic prostatitis.

    Saw Palmetto extract has been extensively studied as a treatment for lower urinary tract symptoms or LUTS. LUTS is a broad umbrella term for pain and urination symptoms associated with BPH, chronic prostatitis, OAB, and IC/PBS, but it's most often

Chapter 5
Supplements for Chronic Prostatitis

used with BPH. Since the 1990s, there have been 58 RCT studies of saw palmetto extract for the treatment of LUTS, with a total of 13,066 patients that ranged from three months to 180 months, with most studies lasting 6 to 12 months. All but three of the studies reported significant improvement in urinary symptoms and quality of life, including an average improvement in IPSS scores of 36%, 34% in quality-of-life scores, and 26% in QMAX or maximum urinary flow rate. The vast majority of these studies were done in Europe and Asia and used a verified LSESr saw palmetto with 85% fatty acids made by pharmaceutical companies. (11)

My experience with flower pollen extract and saw palmetto extract is consistent with the research on the five core phytotherapy treatments for chronic prostatitis. The research shows that flower pollen extract is the most effective treatment for chronic prostatitis, and in my case, it was, in fact, the single most effective treatment. Once again, consistent with the research, saw palmetto proved to be the second most effective treatment for my chronic prostatitis symptoms. It's important to caution, as I have throughout this book that your individual experience may be different, and, in your case, PSO, NRE, or Quercetin may prove to be more effective in flower pollen or saw palemetto.

Dosages and Brands

Studies show that the optimal dosage of saw palmetto extract is 320 mg. Almost all studies on chronic prostatitis and LUTS have used this standard dosage. A few studies have tried a dosage as high as 960 mg and found no additional benefit, and at the same time, no additional adverse side effects have been reported from a dosage as high as 960 mg. The one product that is available in the US that is USP certified and proven in a study of 28 different brands to meet the LSESr 85% fatty acid standard is Flowmentum ®. The most widely used and studied LSESr saw palmetto extract in Europe and Asia; Permixon, a pharmaceutical company in France, manufactures it, but it is not available in the US. There is every reason to believe that because Flowmentum is an 85% fatty acid LSESr saw palmetto just like Permixon, your results will be comparable to the results reported in studies of Permixon. In fact, in my case, while in France, I purchased a 60-day supply of Permixon and found that Flowmentum was actually more effective than Permixon.

Combination Treatments

Saw Palmetto with Nettle Root & Pycnogenol

The nettle root extract has been studied alone and in combination as a treatment for LUTS, which is mostly related to BPH. There is less research about nettle root alone or in combination as a treatment specifically for chronic prostatitis. A 2007 study by Pavone and colleagues is interesting because it was a long-term study that involved a relatively large number of men and reported a substantial improvement in symptoms. In this RCT study, 320 men with a 50/50 mix of chronic prostatitis and BPH received either a placebo or a combination of 320 milligrams of saw palmetto, 120 milligrams of nettle root extract, and 5 milligrams of pycnogenol for 1 year. The combination treatment group showed an 85% improvement in symptoms. The greatest areas of benefit were pain, nighttime urination, and urgency. (12) In this study, nettle root extract and pycnogenol enhanced the pain reduction and urination symptom improvement of saw palmetto extract for chronic prostatitis patients. Unfortunately, with only one study, we don't have enough scientific research to justify it as a recommended standard therapy, especially

Chapter 5
Supplements for Chronic Prostatitis

because pycnogenol is expensive and lacks research as a standalone treatment for chronic prostatitis.

Saw Palmetto with Lycopene & Selenium

A study by Morgia et al. for chronic prostatitis compared LSESr saw palmetto combined with lycopene and selenium (Profluss) to LSESr saw palmetto alone. After eight weeks, the Profluss group saw a 51.64% reduction in symptoms compared to a 26.06% reduction for the saw palmetto-only group. Lycopene and selenium have both been studied separately and shown to provide some limited benefit for prostate health. While this is only one study, and the study period was too short, it provides some limited evidence that adding lycopene and selenium to saw palmetto may enhance its benefits. (13) If you see some improvement with saw palmetto, it may be worthwhile to experiment with adding lycopene and selenium for three months to determine if they can enhance your results from saw palmetto, especially because both of them are inexpensive and research shows that they can help with chronic prostatitis symptoms as standalone treatments.

Saw Palmetto with B Vitamins & Folic Acid

There have been 5 studies done during the past 10 years of Deprox 500, which is a combination of 500 mg of saw palmetto with vitamins B1, B2, B6, B12, and folic acid. Deprox is made by a pharmaceutical company in Italy. These studies compared Deprox to ibuprofen and saw Palmetto extract alone, as well as bromelain and quercetin. Deprox was substantially more effective in all these studies. In 4 RCT studies, the percentage of men reporting a 25% improvement or better in total CPSI scores ranged from 75% to 84% for Deprox. One study is particularly interesting because they compared Deprox to saw palmetto alone. In a 6-week 2019 study by

Macchione and colleagues, 84% of the Deprox group reported a 25% or better improvement in total CPSI scores compared to 65% for saw palmetto. **(14)** This 6-week study suggests that adding B vitamins and folic acid can result in making saw palmetto more effective faster, but we can't draw any conclusions from this 6-week study about the long-term benefit.

Saw Palmetto & Nettle Root Extract

There have been several studies on the combination of saw palmetto with nettle root extract as a treatment for LUTS symptoms primarily associated with BPH. The results of these studies suggest that this combination may also be beneficial, particularly for the urination symptoms of chronic prostatitis. A meta-analysis done by Kirscher-Hermanns and colleagues in 2019 reviewed the results of 4 RCT studies in 960 men with LUTS That compared a combination of 160 milligrams of saw Palmetto and 120 milligrams of nettle root extract taken twice a day in a product called Prostagutt ® Forte made by a pharmaceutical company in Germany. The four studies ranged from 24 to 60 weeks, and the combination of placebo in two of the studies, finasteride in one study, and Tamsulosin in another study was compared. The men taking the saw palmetto abstract/nettle root extract combination saw a 52.9% improvement in their total IPSS scores, with the scores for men with moderate LUTS improving 45.2% and those with severe LUTS improving 88.5% compared to just 6.4% and 11.5% in the placebo group respectively. The results were comparable when compared to the finasteride or tamsulosin group but without the serious side effects that many men experience with these two prescription drugs. (15) I discuss nettle root extract as one of the five core Prostatitis 360 protocol supplements for the treatment of urination symptoms, particularly in the chapter on urination symptoms.

Chapter 5
Supplements for Chronic Prostatitis

Quercetin

Quercetin has been studied and used for the treatment of chronic prostatitis since the 1990s. Most of the research has been done in the US and Canada by two of the most prominent chronic prostatitis researchers in North America. Quercetin is an anti-inflammatory and antioxidant bioflavonoid found in several foods, including grapes, tea, onions, red wine, and citrus fruits, among others. The normal daily dose is 500 mg, but 1000 mg is widely used in scientific studies. It is often included in a wide range of multi-supplement formulations for prostate health, and often, those formulations use less than 500 milligrams. There was no evidence that these products work for BPH or chronic prostatitis. The only proven dose of quercetin is 500mg, and most studies have used 1,000 mg per day.

Scientific Research

In terms of scientific research, there are three key issues with quercetin. There are fewer RCT and non-RCT studies on quercetin for the treatment of both BPH and chronic prostatitis. The few studies that do exist indicate that, on average, quercetin alone is not as effective as the other two major phytotherapies, pollen and saw palmetto, for chronic prostatitis. The studies done have been short, typically 4 weeks, compared to 12 weeks for pollen and saw palmetto, and there are no long-term scientific studies of quercetin. In terms of both the number of studies and the level of evidence of effectiveness, flower pollen and saw palmetto are superior to quercetin. Despite these limitations, it has still proven to be more effective than many pharmaceutical drugs prescribed by urologists to treat chronic prostatitis without the potentially serious side effects of prescription drugs. It's also important to note that most of the quercetin research has been done by two of the most prominent urologists and medical researchers in the field of chronic prostatitis in North America: Dr. J Curtis Nickel at the University of Toronto and Dr. Daniel Shoskes at the Cleveland Clinic.

In a 1999 RCT study done by Shoskes and colleagues using 500 mg of quercetin twice a day for 30 days found that 67% of the patients experienced at least a 25% improvement, and the average improvement was 35% in the quercetin group and 7.2% in the placebo group. Studies show that quercetin is not well absorbed by the human body. This is a major drawback compared to flower pollen and saw palmetto. Bromelain, an extract derived from pineapples, is believed to enhance the absorption of quercetin. In fact, quercetin is often sold with bromelain added to enhance absorption. In a follow-up study by Dr. Shoskes, he used a product called Prosta-Q made by Farr Labs, LLC in Los Angeles, CA, that combines quercetin with cranberry, saw palmetto, bromelain, and papain. In this study, 82% of the patients had at least a 25% improvement. The Prosta-Q product is a "proprietary blend" that totals 540 milligrams. Therefore, we don't know the exact amount of quercetin or the other ingredients used. **(16)** In a 2010 RC T study done by Dr Shoskes using the multimodal UPOINT System, three therapies were selected, including alpha-blockers, physical therapy, and quercetin for a group of 100 patients with CP/CPPS. Alpha-blockers were used for urination symptoms, physical therapy was used for pelvic floor function, and quercetin was used for prostatitis pain. After eight weeks, the quercetin phytotherapy was the single most effective treatment, with the patients who took quercetin reporting a 50% improvement. **(17)** In a 2008 meta-analysis of RCT and non-RCT studies done by Nickel and colleagues, the researchers reviewed 15 nutraceuticals as potential treatments that have been

Chapter 5
Supplements for Chronic Prostatitis

scientifically studied for chronic prostatitis, BPH, and related prostate health conditions. They concluded that saw palmetto, pollen extract, and quercetin had the most rigorous scientific research and the best evidence of effectiveness to recommend them to patients and urologists as treatments for chronic prostatitis. **(18)** A meta-analysis done by Dr. Nickel compared alpha-blockers and quercetin with the treatment of chronic prostatitis. There were 12 widely used alpha blockers studied for six months or longer. Only one, Alfuzosin, was significantly above a 50% response rate of at least 25%. The response rate for eight of them was either below 25% or just above, and two more were in the 50% range. None of the alpha-blockers matched the response 67% rate of quercetin. This is particularly significant because the alpha blockers were typically studied for six months, while quercetin was only studied for one month in most cases. Therefore, while quercetin has the weakest overall benefit of the three scientifically proven psychotherapies for chronic prostatitis, it is still superior to the alpha-blockers commonly prescribed by urologists as of this study. **(19)**

Quercetin vs. Saw Palmetto & Pollen

I believe the best overall conclusion we can make about quercetin, given the limitations of the scientific research and the available results about its effectiveness, is that pollen extract and saw palmetto are the best phytotherapies for chronic prostatitis. However, I believe it's important to include quercetin in your treatment protocol. In my case, the question provided a very small but measurable improvement in my pain symptoms and made a meaningful improvement in the quality of my life. The three proven nutraceuticals are similar but also different enough that for some men, quercetin may be the most effective therapy. And there is enough scientific data to support that possibility. In short, for some men, even if it's a small percentage of men, the best option may turn out to be quercetin. If you don't try quercetin, you may miss out on the best phytotherapy treatment for you.

As for pollen and saw palmetto, long-term studies show that pollen extract is the only supplement that can provide a cure for 20% to 46% of men studied for six months or longer. However, the mechanisms by which they work are different enough that most men should use both, and some men will find that saw palmetto is more effective as part of the complete Prostatitis 360 Protocol.

While some of the three may work better than the others in your case, I believe that taking all three is the best strategy. I believe most men will benefit from all three, but the level of benefit will vary among the three. I think that it's likely that there is a synergistic effect when you take all three phytotherapies. In other words, it's more likely that you will see a greater benefit from one of the phytotherapy supplements if you take the other two. All the major Prostatitis 360 Protocol treatment components, including diet, lifestyle, the three phytotherapies, and the other nutraceuticals, work in different ways to lower inflammation and oxidative stress and relax the urethra and bladder. The logical assumption is that as one of these lowers inflammation, it makes it easier for others to lower inflammation as well. I believe this is true, for example, in the case of diet. In my case, prior to implementing the diet change, when I tried pollen extract for 75 days, it was ineffective, but after I implemented the Prostatitis 360 anti-inflammation diet, I saw a significant improvement in my symptoms 45 days after starting the pollen extract again. That's why I argue throughout the book that the Prostatitis 360 diet is the foundation on which you build the rest of the protocol, including the three key phytotherapies.

Chapter 5
Supplements for Chronic Prostatitis

Combination Treatments

Quercetin, Lycopene and Curcumin Combinations
Several recent studies in China have focused on lycopene as a potential treatment for chronic prostatitis. A recent rat study found that quercetin and curcumin are more effective when combined with lycopene than either quercetin or curcumin alone. Human trials are currently underway.

Bromelain and Quercetin
Studies show that quercetin is not well absorbed. There is some limited evidence that bromelain may enhance the absorption and effectiveness of quercetin. Several supplement brands, as seen below, sell quercetin and bromelain combinations.

Dosage and Brands
Unlike flower pollen and saw palmetto, where the optimal dosage is well-defined and the best available brands in the US are clear, the optimal dosage and the best brand choices are less clear in the case of quercetin. Most studies have used 500 milligrams taken twice a day or a total of 1,000 mg a day for up to 12 weeks. There are no long-term studies based on the available research on the safety and effectiveness of quercetin for chronic prostatitis. Very high doses can cause liver damage. It is recommended as a precaution that you take a 10-day break from quercetin every 90 days. Several established brands in the US sell 500 milligrams of quercetin, including NOW, Swanson, and Solaray. Bromelain is believed to enhance the absorption of quercetin. There are two widely available, established brands in the US that sell quercetin and bromelain

combinations. Doctor's Best has a supplement with 500 mg of quercetin and 250 mg of bromelain, and NOW Foods has a supplement with 800 mg of Quercetin and 165 mg of bromelain. There are reports that bromelain can cause mild stomach upset or mild diarrhea, but these side effects are believed to be rare and minor. If you don't experience any digestive side effects, adding bromelain may enhance the benefits of quercetin.

Pumpkin Seed Oil and Nettle Root Extract

Pumpkin seed oil and nettle root extract are primarily used to treat the urination symptoms of chronic prostatitis. Chapter 8, which is dedicated to urination issues, includes a detailed discussion of pumpkin seed oil and nettle root extract as the two most important treatments for urination problems. Studies show that these two phytotherapies effectively treat a wide range of urination issues, including daytime frequency, nighttime nocturia, and urgency. They also significantly improve the quality of life. Pumpkin seed oil has been extensively studied as a standalone treatment for chronic prostatitis. The nettle root extract has been studied as a standalone treatment, but in most studies, it is combined with saw palmetto. It's also important to note that in addition to improving urination symptoms, this phytotherapy can also, in some cases, provide a small but meaningful improvement in pain symptoms directly or indirectly by lowering the perception of pain. In short, while they primarily help with urination symptoms, they also help with pain symptoms.

    These two phytotherapies are for men who need additional help with urination symptoms. This could be for a number of reasons, including urination symptoms being the greater problem all along, the improvement in urination symptoms lagging behind the

Chapter 5
Supplements for Chronic Prostatitis

improvement in pain symptoms using the three core phytotherapy, and attaining an 85% to 95% improvement in both symptoms but needing an additional treatment to reach the cure. For men who need additional help with urination symptoms, these two phytotherapies should be treated as the 4th and 5th core supplement treatments for their chronic prostatitis. This is especially true for men who find that their urination symptoms are more serious or slower to respond to treatment.

Nettle Root Extract

Nettle Root Extract (NRE), also known as Stinging Nettle Root, has been widely used in Europe for over 20 years to treat BPH and chronic prostatitis. In Europe, it's manufactured by pharmaceutical companies, and all the studies discussed below are based on the NRE made by pharmaceutical companies. NRE, as a standalone treatment, has been shown to be effective in treating urination symptoms in several studies.

A particularly interesting 6-month double-blind placebo-controlled RCT study done in 2005 by Safari Nejad and colleagues with 588 patients who took 500 mg of NRE reported significant improvement in 81% of the patients in the NRE group compared to 16% for the placebo group. Overall urination symptoms, as measured by IPSS, the International Prostate Symptom Score, improved by 40% for the NRE group compared to just 7% for the placebo group. The peak flow rate improved by 8.2 mL/s for the NRE group compared to 3.4 mL/s for the placebo group. This is a significant improvement for the NRE group. The peak flow rate for men typically ranges from 10 to 20 mL/s. A peak flow rate of 15 m/Ls is considered normal. The peak flow rate is a measure of the strength or weakness of urine flow. A weak urine stream is a common symptom of urination problems. A follow-up done 18 months after the study showed that the improvements achieved in the study remained in place for those men who continued treatment with NRE, and most men chose to continue the treatment. None of the men in the study reported any significant side effects. **(20)**

However, most of the high-quality studies with NRE have combined NRE & SPE. A 2019 study by Kirschner-Hermann and colleagues compared the combination of SPE and NRE to two commonly used prescription drugs, Finasteride and Tamsulosin. The study used 160 mg of SPE and 120 milligrams of NRE taken twice daily. The SPE & NRE combination was significantly better than the placebo in treating urination symptoms with no side effects reported and comparable to Finasteride and Tamsulosin, both of which have serious potential side effects and are often discontinued due to side effects the patients can't tolerate, especially after long-term use. **(21)**

Nocturia, waking up two or more times to urinate during sleep, is a particularly problematic urination symptom for men with chronic prostatitis. The poor sleep caused by nocturia is believed to negatively impact immune health, gut health, and depression, which in turn directly or indirectly negatively impact chronic prostatitis symptoms. Studies show that the combination of SPE &NRE can improve nocturia symptoms. The study done by Oelke and colleagues in 2014 with 922 patients who took one 120 mg NRE and 160 mg of SPE twice a day for 24 weeks saw a 50% improvement versus placebo in their nocturia symptoms with nighttime urination declining from an average of 2.1 to 1 per night. The study also compared the NRE and SPE combination with the commonly used drugs Finasteride and Tamsulosin and reported comparable results without the potentially serious side effects of those two drugs. **(22)**

A common objection to nutraceuticals like SPE and an NRE is that, in some cases, there is a lack of long-term studies to determine

Chapter 5
Supplements for Chronic Prostatitis

how effective they are after 6 or 12 months. However, in the case of SPE & NRE, there are long-term studies. A long-term study conducted by Lopatkin and colleagues, for example, published in 2007, involved 257 men who took 120 milligrams of NRE and 160 milligrams of SPE twice a day for 96 weeks. After 24 weeks, the researchers reported 53% lower IPSS scores, a 19% improvement in peak urinary flow, and a 44% decrease in residual urine volume in the bladder. These improvements were significantly better than those of the placebo after 24 weeks. The improvements held steady after 48 weeks and 96 weeks. **(23)** There is, in short, compelling scientific evidence that adding nettle root extract to the Prostatitis 360 phytotherapy treatment protocol that includes Saw Palmetto can significantly improve most urination symptoms.

Dosage and Brands

The typical dosage used in studies in Europe has been 120 milligrams taken twice a day. In the US, NRE is sold in much higher doses. The NOW brand sells a 250 mg version, and Swanson has a 500 mg version of NRE, both of which are good options. Most other US brands sell NRE with 1,000 mg or more. In my case, I take the Swanson 500 mg version once a day, and it has been very effective. There is no evidence that these higher doses are effective, and there was no research about the safety of taking high-dose NRE in the long term. It's generally not a good idea to take high doses of any supplement unless it's supported by scientific evidence and has been studied long-term for side effects.

Pumpkin Seed Oil

Pumpkin seed oil (PSO) is believed to be effective in reducing urinary symptoms in part by helping to relax the bladder, decrease the sense of urinary urgency, decrease bladder spasms, and increase bladder capacity. Several rigorous scientific studies done during the past 25 years have reported that pumpkin seed oil (PSO) can significantly improve urination symptoms and quality of life. The level of improvement reported in these studies ranges from a 30% to 46% improvement in urinary symptoms and quality of life. Studies show that NRE is more effective than PSO, but how you respond to each may vary. You may find that PSO is more effective in your case. If NRE doesn't work for you, PSO is another option. As a standalone treatment, PSO is not a cure for these symptoms, nor will it provide a dramatic improvement. A moderate improvement in your urinary symptoms and quality of life can nevertheless have a significant overall impact. If you have seen, for example, a 50% improvement in your urination symptoms by implementing the Prostatitis 360 Protocol, an additional 20% improvement, for example, achieved by adding PSO, can make a significant difference in your symptoms and quality of life. This scenario is just a theoretical example. Your situation and the results you achieve by adding PSO, NRE, and the other nutraceuticals I discuss below will vary.

A study done in 2000 by Friederich and colleagues with 2,245 patients who took 1,000 mg of pumpkin seed oil reported significant improvements after 12 weeks. There was an average 41% reduction in urination symptoms and a 46% improvement in quality of life. Side effects were rare and minor, with 96% of the participants reporting no side effects and 4% reporting minor side effects. **(24)**

Chapter 5
Supplements for Chronic Prostatitis

There's a limited number of studies of nutraceuticals, such as pumpkin seed oil, that focus on OAB. The 2014 study by Nishimura and colleagues focused on OAB symptoms not related to conditions such as BPH and used the OAB symptom scale or OABSS (Overactive Bladder Symptom Score) to analyze the results. In the study, 45 patients took 10,000 mg of PSO for 12 weeks. After 12 weeks, the overall OABSS declined by 4.4 points for the PSO group compared to 2.7 points for the placebo group. The PSO group achieved an overall OABSS reduction of 38%, a 42% reduction in daytime frequency, a 31% reduction in nocturia, and a 93% reduction in urgency. There are, however, two limitations to this study. The dosage used is 10 times higher than most studies of PSO. Most studies use 1,000 mg, and this study used 10,000 mg. The other difference is the variety of pumpkin seed oil used in this study. Most studies in the US and Europe use a variety of PSOs that are known by the scientific name *Cucurbita Pepo*. This study used a variety of PSO commonly harvested in Asia, which is known by the scientific name *Cucurbita Maxima*. This study did not report any significant side effects after 12 weeks, but there is no data on the long-term side effects of taking such a large dose of PSO. We also don't know if the difference in the variety of PSO used had any significant impact on the results reported in the study. **(25)** Another study that focused on OAB used a combination of 87.5% PSO and 12.5% equol soy extract. In this study by Shim and colleagues done in 2014, 120 participants took the PSO soy extract combination for 12 weeks. The researchers used six different symptom measures from the OABSS, including urination frequency, urgency, incontinence frequency, maximum urgency score, nocturia, and the overall OAB symptom score, and reported significant improvements in all six measures of the OAB symptom scale. **(26)** A 2017 study by Leibbrand and colleagues involved 60 men who took 500 milligrams of PSO for three months. The researchers reported a 30% reduction in total IPSS scores as well as significant reductions in nocturia and a significant improvement in the quality-of-life score. **(27)** In 2016, Damiano and colleagues analyzed 6 RCT studies of PSO used for urinary symptoms, including four studies that reported quality-of-life results. The researchers reported that all six studies showed significant improvements in urinary symptoms. The four studies that included quality of life scores also reported significant improvements in quality of life. **(28)**

Dosage and Brands

Most studies of PSO have used a 1,000 mg to 1,500 mg dosage per day. There are three established widely available brands in the US, NOW, Swanson, and Puritan Pride, that sell 1,000 mg of PSO. You can experiment with increasing the daily dose to 2,000 to determine if it's more effective.

Tier 2 Supplements

Additional Supplements for Chronic Prostatitis

The following supplements have important anti-inflammation, immune system, digestive health, and enhanced absorption benefits that will enhance the impact of the five primary phytotherapies. While there is little or no evidence that they are effective as standalone treatments for chronic prostatitis, their role in reducing inflammation and improving the immune system and digestive health can play a role in improving the effectiveness of the Prostatitis 360 Protocol.

Zinc: Zinc is a very important mineral for prostate health. Studies show that a normal prostate has 744 mcg of zinc compared to 476

Chapter 5
Supplements for Chronic Prostatitis

mcg for men with chronic prostatitis. A 12-week study of men with chronic prostatitis who took 220 mg of zinc showed a small but statistically significant improvement in their symptoms. The extremely high dosage of zinc in this study may be too high even if it is only taken for 12 weeks. **(29)** (Gomez, 2007) Several studies have found that Zinc reduces inflammation and improves immune function. In a 2010 study of 40 older adults, for example, those who took 45 mg of zinc per day experienced greater reductions in inflammatory markers than a placebo group. **(30)** (Bao, 2010). Dietary sources of zinc include shellfish, oysters, and red meat. Statins, alcohol, antacids, diuretics, high sugar intake, and diabetes can deplete or interfere with the absorption of zinc. Zinc levels and zinc absorption decline significantly after age 50. If you are over 50, a good approach may be to take 45 to 60 mg of zinc, add dietary sources of zinc, and remove alcohol, antacids, and sugar to improve the absorption of zinc. After 3 to 6 months, it may be wise to step down to 30 mg. Experts advise against taking more than 40 mg long-term. Too much zinc can cause gastrointestinal problems and lower immunity, both of which are important issues for men with chronic prostatitis. Zinc should be balanced with a small amount of copper. The supplement maker NOW sells a zinc supplement called L-OptiZinc® with 30 mg zinc and 0.3 mg copper, which provides this balance.

Vitamin D: A total of 20,000 IU minimum per day and ideally 40,000 IU taken 4x a day divided at breakfast, lunch, dinner, and bedtime. Vitamin D levels begin to decline significantly after age 40. Vitamin D is one of the most powerful antioxidant supplements. It performs a wide range of critical functions in the body to prevent many forms of inflammation from occurring in the first place. This is in contrast to anti-inflammatories, which, depending on how powerful they are, can significantly reduce inflammation but not entirely eliminate or prevent it. A combination of both is necessary to manage inflammation in the body, including the prostate. In addition to a vitamin D supplement, it is important to obtain vitamin D from regular exposure to the sun. Zinc and vitamins C and D are important in building and maintaining a strong immune system, which is important for men with chronic prostatitis.

Melatonin: 5 mg of a time-released version taken 1 hour before bedtime. In addition to helping with the quality and duration of sleep, which is important for immune health, new research indicates that melatonin is also a very powerful antioxidant comparable to vitamin D, with a wide range of important benefits, including improving the immune system, lowering inflammation, and reducing pain. Several recent studies using mice have shown that melatonin lowers inflammation and could be a potential treatment for chronic prostatitis. This research is still preliminary; so far, no human studies have been conducted. A 5mg time-released version of melatonin taken 1 hour before bedtime may be ideal for most men with chronic prostatitis. The supplement maker Natrol has 5mg and 3mg versions of melatonin that are time-released.

Vitamin C: Vitamin C is a powerful anti-inflammatory. However, vitamin C supplements can irritate the bladder and worsen urination symptoms for a man with chronic prostatitis. Dietary sources of vitamin C do not irritate the bladder and are the best way to obtain vitamin C. Broccoli and cauliflower, for example, are excellent sources of vitamin C and should be added to the daily diet of men with chronic prostatitis.

Chapter 5
Supplements for Chronic Prostatitis

Probiotics: One or two tablets of a basic probiotic with 10 to 14 strains and a total of 25 to 35 billion CFU is adequate for most men after completing the first 90 days of the anti-inflammation diet. If, however, you have a history of IBS, acid reflux, ulcers, or other digestive tract issues, you should take a probiotic with more strains that are focused specifically on digestion. Most makers of probiotics offer a digestion formula. These probiotics are very expensive. The probiotic maker Garden of Life has a product called Prostate +, which promotes probiotics for prostate, digestive, and immune system health at approximately $50 for a 30-day supply. Once you implement the anti-inflammation diet and see significant improvement in your digestive issues, you can downgrade to a less expensive probiotic. The anti-inflammation diet will, in most cases, have the greatest single impact on the health of your digestive system, but probiotics should remain a part of the core daily supplement regimen to complement the wide variety of prebiotic foods in the anti-inflammation diet. Our digestive system needs a good mix of prebiotic and probiotic ingredients for maximum health. Unfortunately, almost all probiotic foods are restricted to the anti-inflammation diet. Therefore, a daily probiotic supplement remains necessary in the long term. One option for an inexpensive basic probiotic from a widely available established brand is Probiotic-10 25 billion from NOW Foods.

Bioperine: Bioperine 10 mg per day in the morning enhances the absorption of all supplements. This can be particularly beneficial for men over 60 because the absorption of many supplements starts to decline after 50 and is more severe after 60. However, if you are taking any prescription drugs, you should be cautious because bioperine can also enhance the absorption of some prescription drugs. If you are taking a prescription drug, as always, discuss this supplement with your doctor and work with your doctor to carefully monitor the level of any drug in your system on a regular basis.

Potential Future Supplement for Chronic Prostatitis

The following are two groups of supplements. The first group consists of supplements that have been studied for the treatment of chronic prostatitis, and the second group consists of supplements that have been studied primarily for the treatment of BPH. If there is rigorous scientific research in the future for treating chronic prostatitis, some of these may emerge as important for combination, secondary, and add-on treatments for chronic prostatitis or perhaps a new major supplement therapy.

Nutraceuticals Studied for Chronic Prostatitis

There are several nutraceuticals that have been studied for the treatment of chronic prostatitis symptoms In addition to the three major proven treatments. All these nutraceuticals will require a great deal more research before we can make any meaningful judgments about their potential to be significant additional treatment options for men with chronic prostatitis. These nutraceuticals include the following:

> **Lycopene**: Lycopene has been studied in three recent rat studies as a stand-alone treatment for chronic prostatitis. A human study discussed above under saw palmetto that combined lycopene and selenium with saw palmetto significantly enhanced the benefits of saw palmetto. There is ongoing lycopene research in China, including human studies. We may know in the next five years how significant lycopene will be in the treatment of chronic prostatitis symptoms. A 2013 human RCT study done by Lombardo and

colleagues in Italy studied the combination of lycopene, selenium, and zinc and found it significantly lowered the CPSI pain scores of men with chronic prostatitis. **(31)** It remains to be seen whether lycopene will emerge in the future as a significant new treatment for chronic prostatitis, standalone or in combination with other supplements.

Berberine: Berberine has been studied in China. A 2019 meta-analysis of 21 studies by Hui-Juan and colleagues involved 3359 patients diagnosed with chronic prostatitis. The patients were given a product called Prostant in the form of a daily suppository. The main ingredient of Prostant is berberine. The researchers reported that the Prostant group had significant improvements in pain, urination symptoms, and quality of life. Twice as many of the patients in the Prostant group reported improvement as the placebo group. The researchers also concluded that more rigorous scientific studies are necessary. More RCT studies are ongoing and planned in China. The initial very limited results are promising, and berberine may emerge as a significant treatment option in the future. These studies done in China will also have to be replicated in studies done outside of China. **(32)**

N-Acetyl Cysteine or NAC: There have been two studies of NAC, a rat study done in China and a human study in Russia, and both showed promising results. In the human study in 2020 done by Gorpynchenko and colleagues, 60 patients were divided into two groups. Group 1 was treated with 1000 milligrams of quercetin for 120 days, and Group 2 was treated with 600 milligrams of NAC. The researchers reported that 63% of the patients in the NAC group saw at least a 25% improvement. While impressive, this did not match the results reported by the quercetin group. **(33)** There must be a great deal more research on NAC before we can make any judgments about its potential to treat chronic prostatitis symptoms. Nevertheless, the initial research is promising. The Gorpynchenko study was only a 12-week study. It often takes up to six months to see the full impact of a supplement. Long-term studies are needed before we can make any conclusive judgments about NAC.

General Note of Caution: The review above of the limited number of studies for these nutraceuticals is based on widely available studies done in English or translated into English. While most scientific research done around the world is reported in English, it is possible that there have been studies done in China, Russia, or Japan, for example, that have not been translated and are not easily accessible to readers and researchers outside of those countries. It is, therefore, possible that additional research has been done on the nutraceuticals discussed above that have not been included in this review.

BPH and Chronic Prostatitis

There is a significant overlap in the symptoms and the treatments for chronic prostatitis and BPH. The best illustration of this overlap is saw palmetto, which has been extensively studied, proven to be effective, and widely used in Europe to treat both chronic prostatitis and BPH. Since urinary symptoms are the primary symptoms of BPH the supplements used to treat BPH also primarily target urination symptoms. Chapter 8 is dedicated to treating persistent urination symptoms that don't fully respond to the five core chronic prostatitis supplements as part of the Prostatitis 360 Protocol. It includes a detailed review of nettle root extract and pumpkin seed oil for the treatment of the urination symptoms of chronic prostatitis.

Saw palmetto, nettle root extract, and pumpkin seed oil are widely used in Europe as first-line treatments for BPH. In Germany, Austria, and France, these phytotherapies led by saw palmetto account for up to 50% of the prescriptions written for BPH. The success of these three supplements in treating the urination symptoms of BPH indirectly supports their potential for treating the urination symptoms of chronic prostatitis. Several other nutraceuticals have been studied and, to varying degrees, used to treat BPH, primarily in Europe, including Pygeum Africanum, Beta-sitosterol, African plum tree, and South African star grass, among others. However, BPH-related research is limited, and there is no significant scientific evidence that they are effective for chronic prostatitis.

Implementing The Chronic Prostatitis 360 Phytotherapy Protocol

Three-Part Implementation Plan

The first step in implementing the phytotherapy protocol is actually not to start taking the supplements but to start by implementing the Prostatitis 360 Anti-Inflammation Diet for a minimum of 60 days and ideally 90 days before you start taking the supplements.

A. Diet: Implement the Prostatitis 360 anti-inflammation diet

   1. Start by removing all alcohol, caffeine, and spicy foods.
   2. Implement the rest of the diet as quickly as you can.
   3. Read Chapter 4 for a step-by-step guide to implementing the diet.

B. Supplements: Take the 5 core Tier 1 phototherapies

   1. Flower pollen extract: 500 mg taken at breakfast, lunch, and dinner for a total of 1500 mg daily. Product: Pollen Aid made by Germinex, LLC.
   2. LSESr saw palmetto: 320 mg daily in the morning with breakfast. Product: Flowmentum distributed by Flowmentum Health
   3. Quercetin: 500 mg taken at lunch and dinner for a total of 1000 mg daily. Product: NOW, Swanson, and Soloray are widely available, established brands that sell 500 mg of quercetin.
   4. Pumpkin seed oil: 1000 mg daily. Product: NOW, Swanson and Puritan Pride
   5. Nettle root extract: 500 mg daily. Product: NOW and Swanson

C. Supplements: Gradually phase in the remaining secondary and add-on supplements. For most men, steps 1 through 4 below should be part of the daily supplement program. Steps 5 and 6 are optional based on your individual needs and experience.

   1. Digestive probiotics to help improve your overall digestive system
   2. Melatonin to improve sleep quality, especially if you have nocturia
   3. Bioperine to enhance the absorption of all the supplements
   4. Take zinc and vitamin D, and add more C from your diet

Chapter 5
Supplements for Chronic Prostatitis

5. Add selenium and lycopene to enhance the effectiveness of saw palmetto if necessary
6. Add B vitamins and folic acid to enhance the effectiveness of saw palmetto as another option

Diet and the Synergistic Effect of the Protocol

While some of the five core supplements may work better than the others in your case, I believe that all of the above approaches are the best strategies. I believe most men will see benefits from all five, but the level of benefit will vary among the five. I think that it is likely that there is a synergistic effect when you take all five phytotherapies. In other words, it is more likely that you will see a greater benefit from one of the phytotherapy supplements if you take the other four. All the major Prostatitis 360 Protocol treatment components, including diet, lifestyle, the five phytotherapies, and the other nutraceuticals, work in different ways and to varying degrees to lower inflammation and oxidative stress. I believe that as one of these lowers inflammation, it makes it easier for others to lower inflammation. This is particularly true in the case of diet.

The primary focus of this chapter is a nutraceutical protocol for treating the symptoms of chronic prostatitis. In the process, we have addressed the two dominant symptoms of chronic prostatitis: pain and urination. However, there are two other major symptoms, sexual side effects, and depression, that also impact most men with chronic prostatitis. In chapter 9, I focus on the sexual side effects, and in chapter 10, I focus on depression and stress management. I will review a wide range of therapy strategies for depression and sexual side effects, including diet, nutraceuticals, and lifestyle treatments, as well as specific conventional medical treatments and drug therapies.

CHAPTER 6
Chronic Prostatitis Lifestyle Changes

While lifestyle changes and their impact on chronic prostatitis symptoms have not been as extensively studied as supplements, compelling research done in the past 20 years shows that lifestyle changes can significantly improve the symptoms of chronic prostatitis.

The most comprehensive study to date on the impact of diet and lifestyle changes on chronic prostatitis was done in Italy by Gallo and colleagues in 2014. **(1)** The study divided 100 men diagnosed with chronic prostatitis into two groups. Group one took 100mg of INSAID per day, and group 2 followed a protocol of 13 diet and lifestyle changes plus one 100mg of INSAID per day. The 13 diet and lifestyle changes were selected based on extensive prior research that showed they were effective in lowering the symptoms of chronic prostatitis. After three months, group 2 reported a dramatic reduction in average CPSI scores with a drop from 20.1 to 8.1 or a 60% overall reduction in chronic prostatitis symptoms. There were also similar improvements in specific

CHAPTER 6
Chronic Prostatitis Lifestyle Changes

subcategories, such as pain and urination symptoms. The drop in average CPSI scores for the placebo group one was relatively modest, with an average reduction from 21.9 to 17.6. The study highlights one of the challenges of some of the lifestyle changes necessary to improve chronic prostatitis symptoms. Abstaining from alcohol is particularly difficult for many men, and collectively, the 13 changes in the study add up to a dramatic diet and lifestyle change for most men. This is highlighted by the fact that there was a 22% dropout rate in the study. I believe, however, that men struggling with severe long-term chronic prostatitis symptoms will, in most cases, decide to make these dramatic changes. The 13 changes organized by category are:

A. Dietary Changes

1. Alcohol
   The consumption of alcohol has consistently been shown in numerous studies over the past 30 years to have the greatest direct connection with chronic prostatitis symptoms, including studies that show consuming more alcohol results in more severe symptoms. In short, alcohol consumption is the single most important of these 13 lifestyle changes. This involves completely abstaining from all forms of alcohol, including beer, wine, and champagne.

2. Caffeine
   Abstaining from all forms of caffeine and coffee, including decaffeinated coffee and tea. Caffeine is found in a wide range of other foods in addition to coffee, such as cola, soft drinks, and all forms of chocolate. Caffeine-free herbal teas and white chocolate are suitable alternatives. Studies show

that caffeine makes voiding symptoms worse and causes muscle spasms in men with chronic pelvic pain.

3. Spicy Foods
The following spicy foods should be removed from the diet: hot peppers, hot sauce, chilis, horseradish, and most Mexican, Thai, and Indian foods. These spicy foods are associated with urination symptoms and may cause more severe urination symptoms.

4. Dietary Mix Changes
Studies show that a diet high in carbohydrates, low in fruits and vegetables, and high in milk-related products, including cheese, is associated with a greater likelihood of chronic prostatitis symptoms. The recommended diet includes a lower consumption of carbohydrates, eliminating milk-related products, and significantly increasing consumption of fruits and vegetables.

5. Bowel Disorders
Studies show a strong association between chronic constipation, diarrhea, abdominal pain and swelling, and chronic prostatitis symptoms. The recommended diet changes include increasing fruits and vegetables significantly and adopting a high-fiber diet, including pure psyllium and oatmeal. Aerobic exercise and stress management can also help.

B. Sexual Habits
1. Avoid delaying ejaculation. Delaying ejaculation may cause pelvic muscle spasms.

CHAPTER 6
Chronic Prostatitis Lifestyle Changes

2. Avoid sexual abstinence. The recommended weekly frequency is a minimum of twice a week.
3. Avoid excessive ejaculation. Two or more per day is excessive.
4. Do not practice coitus interruptus as a means of family planning. It may cause swelling of the prostate.

C. Lifestyle

Sedentary lifestyle.

Studies show that a sedentary lifestyle is associated with a greater risk of chronic prostatitis. Several studies also show that regular exercise, especially aerobic exercise, can improve the symptoms of chronic prostatitis. The recommended aerobic exercise program is 30 to 45 minutes of walking, jogging, or swimming four times a week.

D. Pelvic Floor Muscle Trauma.

The following are applicable to chronic prostatitis but may be particularly relevant for chronic pelvic pain patients.

1. Sitting too long
   Sitting for long periods is strange to the pelvic floor muscles. If you must sit for long periods, the recommendation is to use a donut-shaped cushion and, if possible, a standing desk.
2. Sports that cause pelvic floor strain
   Avoid sports such as cycling, rowing, horseback riding, motorcycle riding, etc., that strain the pelvic floor muscle area. Some forms of weightlifting may also strain the pelvic floor area.

3. Tight Clothing
   Tight clothing in the pelvic area is associated with a higher risk of symptoms in IC patients. It is not clear how relevant this is for chronic prostatitis patients.

The Gallo study ranks the 13 changes by how important they were in the study outcome. The rankings are:

Caffeine:	67
Alcohol:	61
Excessive sex:	58
Coitus interruptus:	47
Bowel disorder:	46
Delay ejaculation:	41
Sexual abstinence:	40
Sedentary life:	36
Sitting too long:	25
Spicey foods:	24
High carb diet:	23
Tight clothing:	23

This is just one ranking. Other studies show different results. Alcohol is often well ahead of other lifestyle factors. Several other important lifestyle modifications are not included in this Gallo study, most notably the role of relaxation techniques and meditation. Stress management is very important for both chronic prostatitis and pelvic floor dysfunction.

The 13 Gallo lifestyle modifications don't exist in a vacuum. Once implemented, they have a wide range of long-term benefits that

Chronic Prostatitis Lifestyle Changes

impact blood pressure, digestive health, borderline diabetes, stress, mental health, and more. All of these, in turn, impact the symptoms of chronic prostatitis. These long-term benefits are not immediately captured in the results of a 90-day study. It may take 6 to 12 months to see the full benefit of this lifestyle, as well as the diet changes and supplements that make up the entire Prostatitis 360 Protocol. It's important to recognize that high blood pressure, diabetes, heart disease, and high cholesterol are serious medical conditions. The Gallo lifestyle changes and the other components of the Prostatitis 360 Protocol can be part of a treatment program for these serious conditions, but they require a complete treatment plan by a medical professional. And in fact, working with your doctor to address these serious conditions is part of the Prostatitis 360 Protocol.

Exercise

In addition to diet changes, exercise has been studied extensively as a standalone treatment for chronic prostatitis. This research shows that aerobic exercise can significantly lower the symptoms of chronic prostatitis. Basic strength training, such as push-ups, sit-ups, and stretching exercises, also provides some, but limited, benefits.

An 18-week study done by Guibilei et al. of 231 men compared an aerobic exercise group to a strength training group, which, in effect, acted as the placebo group. (2) While both the aerobic and strength groups saw improvement, the improvement was much greater in the case of the aerobic group, with significant symptom reductions in overall CPSI scores as well as the pain, quality of life, and urination symptom scores.

A large-scale population study done by Zhang et al. in 2015 evaluated the association between regular exercise and the likelihood of developing chronic prostatitis. This long-term study of over 20,000 men between 40 and 70 years old determined that men who exercise regularly, regardless of the level of intensity, were less likely to develop chronic prostatitis.

Stress Management

Yoga

Yoga is recognized as a form of mind-body complementary and alternative medicine (CAM) that integrates an individual's physical, mental, and spiritual components to improve health, particularly stress-related illnesses. Chronic pelvic pain is believed to be primarily a stress-driven condition, but chronic prostatitis patients can also benefit from stress management techniques such as yoga.

The scientific evidence for the value of yoga in managing stress and depression is weak. A 2018 meta-analysis of eight RCT studies of yoga for stress management involving 319 participants showed a small benefit in improving anxiety and depression. (4). However, it is very difficult to conduct rigorous scientific studies of the practice of yoga. It is a recognized CAM treatment, and there is consistent anecdotal evidence that yoga provides a significant level of improvement for individuals with stress and, to a lesser extent, mild depression. I believe that men with chronic prostatitis who are experiencing significant levels of stress and, to

a lesser extent, mild depression should consider yoga as a treatment option.

CHAPTER 6
Chronic Prostatitis Lifestyle Changes

Six Recommended Poses for Stress

The following six yoga poses are recommended as among the best poses for stress management:

1. Downward-facing dog
2. Upward-facing dog
3. Corpse
4. Child's pose
5. Savasana
6. Legs up the wall

You can find videos online with detailed step-by-step instructions on how to perform these poses.

Meditation

Two types of meditation are widely practiced in the US: Transcendental Meditation and mindfulness meditation. Transcendental Meditation has been extensively studied and proven to be effective in treating stress, anxiety, mild depression, and, to a lesser extent, pain. Hundreds of scientific studies have been conducted on the benefits of the Transcendental Meditation program in treating stress and anxiety at more than 200 independent universities and research institutions worldwide over the past 40 years. "Transcendental Meditation benefits from a vast body of 40 years of research showing very powerful long-lasting reductions in stress and sustained improvements in health," according to Norman Rosenthal, MD, prominent psychiatrist, medical researcher, and best-selling author. Several meta-analyses of Transcendental Meditation consistently show "substantial" improvements in stress, anxiety, and mild depression, as well as significant improvements in coping with pain. A study done in 2022 by Joshi et al. showed a 45% reduction in both mild depression and anxiety after two weeks, a 62% reduction in anxiety, and a 58% reduction in mild depression after 3 months. (5)

The scientific evidence for the potential of other types of meditation, including Mindfulness-Based Therapy (MBT), to help with stress, anxiety, depression, and pain is weak to moderate. A meta-analysis done by researchers at Johns Hopkins University of 47 studies involving 3,320 participants showed a moderate improvement in anxiety, depression, and pain symptoms and a low level of improvement in overall anxiety-related quality of life after both 8 weeks, 3 and 6 months. (6) The researchers concluded that the evidence for the benefit of exercise for anxiety, depression, and pain was stronger than MBT meditation. Transcendental Meditation is believed to be twice as effective for anxiety, depression, and pain compared to MBT.

There is, therefore, strong evidence that Transcendental Meditation (TM) can be an important part of the lifestyle treatment protocol for chronic prostatitis and chronic pelvic floor dysfunction. TM generally requires four sessions done by a professional instructor. The cost in the US is typically $400 to $1,000 and is normally not covered by HMO and PPO health plans. The TM technique is very simple. If you can't afford professional training, you may be able to learn TM on your own with free online instructional resources.

Depression

There are several scientifically proven connections between depression and chronic prostatitis. Men with depression are much more likely to develop chronic prostatitis. Men who have

CHAPTER 6
Chronic Prostatitis Lifestyle Changes

depression are more likely to experience more severe symptoms of chronic prostatitis. Chronic pain, the primary symptom of chronic prostatitis, is one of the main causes of depression. Depression is not only associated with emotional and psychological challenges for men with chronic prostatitis but it is also associated with physical signs of higher inflammation (Cytokines). Depression is the second most common disease in the world after heart disease, with 10% of the population affected by the condition. Chronic depression or clinical depression is a serious medical condition that requires professional medical treatment.

There are, however, steps that men with chronic prostatitis can take on their own to treat mild, moderate, or occasional depression. Lifestyle changes are a good place to start. Many of the lifestyle changes that can help with mild depression are already part of the chronic Prostatitis 360 Protocol, including diet, exercise, improved sleep, and meditation. These lifestyle changes alone could make an important contribution to addressing mild depression for many men.

Supplements for Depression

Some of the secondary vitamins and minerals that help with depression, including zinc, vitamin D, melatonin, and L-theanine, are part of the supplement treatment protocol. Several supplements have been scientifically studied and proven to be effective for mild to moderate depression and, in some cases, more effective than prescription medications with fewer side effects. The following supplements have the greatest scientific research to prove their effectiveness in treating mild to moderate depression.

St. John's Wort

St. John's Wort extract has been extensively studied for over 50 years in the treatment of mild to moderate depression. A 2016 meta-analysis of 27 studies done between 1966 and 2015 involving 3,126 participants showed that St. John's Port was as effective as SSRIs in treating mild to moderate depression with significantly fewer serious side effects. SSRIs are a class of prescription medications used to treat depression. (7). Most of the research has studied the safety and efficacy of two different extracts, hyperforin and hypericin, rather than herbs. The research indicates that a dose of 1-3 percent hyperforin taken at 300 mg three times per day and 0.3 percent hypericin at 300 mg three times per day is beneficial. You also want to choose a product that includes all parts of the plant - flower, stem, and leaves. The hyperforin extract is generally considered better than the hypericin extract. St. John's Wort is for the treatment of mild to moderate depression, not for severe depression or bipolar disorder. It should never be taken in conjunction with SSRIs. Discuss the use of St. John's Wort with your doctor if you're taking any other prescription medications. Studies show that St. John's Wort can cause drug interactions with approximately 50% of prescription drugs. The use of this herb requires a great deal of caution. As a precaution, I would avoid using St. John's Wort If you're taking any prescription drugs unless you and your doctor do extensive research on potential drug interactions.

L-Methylfolate

L-Methylfolate is a specific form of folic acid that is proven in several studies to be effective in treating depression stand-alone as well as combined with SSRIs. L-Methylfolate, unlike St John's Wort, can be combined with SSSIs to treat more serious depression. A study by Shelton et al. of 502 patients who added 15 mg of Deplin (a prescription form of L-Methylfolate) with their existing SSRI drug treatments and 52 patients who took Delpin stand-alone reported significant improvement. (8) After 95 days, 67.9% of the patients saw an average 58.2% improvement in their depression symptoms, and 45.7% achieved remission. Deplin is sold by prescription, but it is labeled as a "medical food" and is not a drug. There are no scientific studies of over-the-counter versions of L-Methylfolate. Despite the lack of clear scientific evidence, over-the-counter L-Methylfolate is widely sold and used as a treatment for depression.

SAMe

SAMe is an over-the-counter supplement that has generally proven to be effective and provides moderate to significant improvement in mild to moderate depression symptoms. A 2020 meta-analysis of 11 studies involving 1,011 participants who took SAMe stand-alone and as an add-on therapy for prescription depression medications showed a significant improvement in symptoms as a stand-alone treatment and as a combination treatment. The dosage ranged from 200 milligrams to 3,200 milligrams, with the typical dosage of 1600 milligrams. Side effects were rare, mild, and transient. (9) Studies have shown that increasing the dosage from 1600 milligrams to 3200 milligrams can improve benefits.

Saffron

Saffron is an herb that is available as an over-the-counter supplement in pill form. It has proven effective in several studies for treating stress and anxiety, as well as moderate to severe depression. A meta-analysis of five studies by Hausenblas et al. involving participants with clinical depression showed that taking saffron significantly reduced symptoms of depression. The typical dosage in these studies was 15 mg twice a day for a total of 30 mg daily. Several studies of saffron for anxiety, stress, and moderate (subclinical) depression have shown similar results in treating these conditions using the same dosage.

There are supplements that have been studied for mild to moderate depression, anxiety, and stress, including EPA/Fish Oil, 5HTP, and vitamin B12. However, to date, these studies have been limited and inconclusive. Research on 5HTP has been promising, but there are concerns about potential serious side effects. Several vitamins and minerals are believed to help with mild depression and anxiety, including B complex vitamins, vitamin D, magnesium, and zinc.

Sleep Quality: The Importance of Sleep Quality for Treating Chronic Prostatitis

Sleep quality is an important underlying health issue for men with chronic prostatitis. Sleep quality impacts chronic pain, immune system strength, inflammation, erectile dysfunction, stress, anxiety, and depression. It has not been widely studied as a stand-alone lifestyle factor associated with chronic prostatitis, but it may be one of the most important lifestyle issues impacting chronic prostatitis.

A wide range of risk factors impact the quality of sleep, including lack of regular exercise, regular alcohol use, obesity, poor diet, age, stress, poor sleep habits, and sleep apnea. Many of these underlying causes of poor sleep are addressed in the Chronic Prostatitis 360 Protocol, including exercise, alcohol use, caffeine use, diet, and stress. Many of the diet changes in the Chronic Prostatitis 360 Diet are associated with improved sleep. Studies

CHAPTER 6
Chronic Prostatitis Lifestyle Changes

show that a diet high in fish, fruits, and vegetables improves sleep quality. (11) Individuals over 50 are likely to sleep less as they get older. It is important to take proactive steps to get 7 to 8 hours of sleep after age 50 and not accept shorter, poor-quality sleep as a "normal" part of aging.

Sleep apnea is a common medical disorder in which individuals briefly stop breathing several times per hour throughout the night while sleeping. It is difficult to detect because most individuals are unaware that they have stopped breathing multiple times throughout the night. It's believed that approximately 30% of men have sleep apnea, but because the condition is difficult to detect, the exact percentage is unknown. Chronic snoring, obesity, and regular alcohol use are among the most common risk factors. Symptoms include chronic snoring, morning headaches, tiredness and yawning throughout the day, and poor focus and concentration. While serious chronic snoring and obesity are most often associated with sleep apnea, many individuals with sleep apnea do not snore and are normal weight. If you have any of the symptoms of sleep apnea or if you are over the age of 50, overweight, do not exercise, drink alcohol on a regular basis, or experience chronic stress, an overnight sleep test is the best way to determine if you have sleep apnea and measure the overall quality have your sleep. If you have sleep apnea, a CPAP breathing machine will dramatically improve the quality of your sleep. Your primary care doctor can refer you to a sleep specialist or sleep clinic. Overnight sleep tests and CPAP machines are routinely covered by health insurance.

7 Sleep Habits for Improved Sleep
Good sleep habits are important to your sleep quality and duration. Good sleep habits are important at any age, but they are

particularly important after 40. The following is the Chronic Prostatitis 360 Sleep Habits Protocol:

1. Sleep Schedule. Go to bed and wake up consistently at the same time every night.
2. Sleep environment. Sleep in a cool, dark, and quiet room.
3. Appropriate bedding. Use a comfortable pillow and mattress, especially if you are a side sleeper.
4. Avoid screen time (TV, PC, smartphone, etc.) one hour before bedtime.
5. Limit fluids 3 hours prior to bedtime. This is especially important for men with chronic prostatitis.
6. Daily or occasional naps: Limit naps to 20 to 30 minutes and take him no later than 3:00 PM.
7. Aerobic exercise. In addition to 30 minutes of aerobic exercise four days a week, try to get some form of aerobic exercise every day on your "off" days by using the stairs instead of the elevator, walking during lunch, taking an after-dinner stroll, etc.

4 Key Supplements for Sleep Quality

The primary symptoms of chronic prostatitis pain, frequent nighttime urination, and stress make it particularly difficult for a man suffering from severe chronic prostatitis to get good quality sleep. Chronic prostatitis symptoms impact every aspect of quality sleep, including latency (how quickly you fall asleep), quality, and duration. While the lifestyle changes we've discussed so far in this chapter can help a great deal for men suffering from severe chronic prostatitis, lifestyle changes alone are often not enough. On the other hand, it is important to note that these lifestyle changes are the foundation for making the following sleep supplements more

CHAPTER 6
Chronic Prostatitis Lifestyle Changes

effective. In other words, supplements are not an alternative to the important and, in some cases, difficult lifestyle changes necessary to improve sleep quality successfully. In general, there is a lack of rigorous scientific research on over-the-counter sleep supplements, but the following supplements have the strongest available scientific evidence for improving sleep quality and helping with stress and relaxation.

Melatonin
A time-release dose of 3mg, 5 mg, or 10 mg helps with all three aspects of good sleep: latency, quality, and duration. The evidence is inconclusive, but some reports show that higher doses of melatonin can increase urinary frequency. Therefore, men with chronic prostatitis should start with 3 mg and carefully monitor the symptoms of frequent urination. It is best to take melatonin one hour before bedtime. The supplement maker, NATROL, has 3mg, 5mg, and 10mg time-release versions of melatonin.

L-Theanine
A dose of 200 mg per day, 100 mg in the morning, and 100 mg one hour before bedtime helps with sleep quality, and this is particularly effective for stress and relaxation to sleep better. The effectiveness of L-Theanine is enhanced when it's combined with magnesium. Magnesium is typically combined and balanced with calcium at a ratio of 1,000 mg calcium and 500 mg magnesium. Adding magnesium is optional and is intended for individuals who need more help with stress and relaxation.

Valerian Root
The most frequently studied dose of valerian root is 530 mg per day in pill form. It is also available as a tea. It helps with latency,

sleep quality, and duration. It is particularly effective for anxiety and mild depression.

Magnesium

A dose of 500 mg of magnesium aids sleep quality in part by helping with muscle relaxation, making it particularly important for men with chronic pelvic floor pain as a sleep aid and to help with muscle relaxation of the pelvic floor muscles. Magnesium increases GABA, which is known to have a calming effect. Magnesium combined with melatonin enhances their combined effectiveness.

Sleep: Important Final Note

Chronic poor sleep and insomnia are serious medical conditions that require prompt medical treatment. If you have chronic insomnia, you should see a sleep specialist. Your primary care doctor can refer you to a sleep specialist.

Part III
Advanced Chronic Prostatitis Treatment

CHAPTER 7
Chronic Pain Management

In this chapter, we focus on chronic prostatitis as a chronic pain condition for men who see significant improvement in the chronic prostatitis symptoms after implementing the Prostatitis 360 Protocol but for whom the improvement in pain lags behind improvement in urination symptoms. In other words, this chapter is designed for men needing additional help improving their pain symptoms. The primary focus is on pain as a symptom and the best available tools to treat pain rather than trying to understand and treat the underlying causes of chronic prostatitis pain. What follows is a chronic pain management protocol based on the best available scientific data on chronic prostatitis pain management.

Chronic pain management starts with diet, aerobic exercise, meditation, yoga, and several other lifestyle changes that are already part of the Chronic Prostatitis 360 Protocol. Some of these lifestyle changes impact inflammation, one of the underlying causes of pain, but they also work by changing our perception of pain. Aerobic exercise, for example, produces endorphins, which are hormones

CHAPTER 7
Chronic Pain Management

that are natural painkillers that increase the threshold for pain. Endorphins interact with pain receptors in the brain, which can change our perception of pain. If you have implemented the aerobic exercise component of the chronic prostatitis protocol and are doing 30 minutes of aerobic exercise four times a week, it may be beneficial to gradually work up to 45 minutes five times a week and increase the intensity of the aerobic exercise by, for example, walking or swimming faster to release more endorphins and lower the perception of pain. The overall value of lifestyle changes is limited in treating serious chronic pain. Aerobic exercise, for example, is rated in scientific studies as having a moderate impact on chronic pain. Lifestyle changes can help to some extent, but they are just the starting point for treating serious chronic pain.

The following is a review of natural or alternative and conventional medical treatments for chronic prostatitis pain. The goal is to identify treatments that work for 50% or more of patients and provide close to or higher than a 50% reduction in pain. The primary tool used by medical researchers to measure the effectiveness of treatments for chronic pain is the visual analog scale (VAS) measure of pain intensity, which measures pain and a scale of zero to 10, with zero being no pain and 10 meaning extremely severe pain which is described "as pain is bad as it could possibly be." This is in addition to using the CPSI pain symptom score.

Natural Treatments for Chronic Prostatitis Pain.

There are a few natural treatments for severe chronic pain that have been scientifically proven to be effective. Natural supplements or nutraceuticals are ideal because they are inexpensive, and most of them have rare and minor, if any, side effects. This contrasts with pharmaceutical pain treatments, which often have side effects ranging from serious to extremely serious, addictive, and even potentially deadly opioid treatments.

The most promising natural treatment is Palmitoylethanolamide (PEA). It has been studied for over 20 years for the treatment of chronic pain and, more recently, for chronic prostatitis pain. Several meta-analyses have shown a significant improvement in chronic pain. The most recent meta-analysis done in 2023 involving 11 studies and 774 patients showed that it was "effective" for treating pain and well-tolerated with no major side effects. (1)

PEA has also been extensively studied in combination with polydatin and has demonstrated some very significant reductions in chronic pelvic pain. Polydatin is a form of resveratrol. A 2019 study used a combination of 400 mg of PEA and 40 mg of polydatin for chronic pelvic pain patients. The 90-day study started with 600 milligrams of PEA alone for 10 days, and 400 milligrams of PEA and 40 milligrams of Polydatin were administered two times a day every 12 hours for the remaining 80 days. This study reported a dramatic 64% reduction in overall pelvic pain using the VAS scale, a 36% reduction in dysuria pain, and a significant improvement in overall quality of life.(2) The study used a product called NEVAMAST ® with 400 milligrams of PEA and 40 milligrams of Polydatin from Epitech Group in Italy. NEVAMAST is only available by prescription in Europe. In the US, PEA, PEA, and Polydatin can be purchased as separate over-the-counter supplements without a prescription and combined to create the equivalent combination of PEA and Polydatin. A 2019 six-month study of MEVAMAST for IC/PBS reported a 33% reduction in chronic pain and a significant improvement in urination symptoms. While IC/PBS Is a different condition from chronic prostatitis, the study is relevant because it involves the urethra and the bladder, some of the same parts of the pelvic area as chronic prostatitis. (3)

CHAPTER 7
Chronic Pain Management

These two studies were non-RCT studies, but a meta-analysis of several studies, including RCT studies, also showed significant improvements in pain and quality of life for patients with chronic pain. (3).

Several studies have combined PEA with other supplements such as ALA, saw palmetto, and magnesium and reported significant improvement in chronic prostatitis symptoms. The most promising of these PEA combination treatment studies for chronic prostatitis involved 600 mg of PEA and 320 of saw palmetto. It resulted in a 42% reduction in pain after 4 weeks. (4) There is strong scientific evidence for PEA as the best natural treatment for chronic pain alone or in combination with saw palmetto, which is already one of the five supplements for chronic prostatitis in the Prostatitis 360 Protocol. Research shows that micronized or "ultra" micronized versions of PEA are more effective. A dose of 600 mg may be a good place to start. Studies have used anywhere from 300 mg to 1,200 mg, with several studies using 600 mg 2 times a day. An important advantage of PEA is that it has minor, if any, side effects. Most pharmaceutical treatments for pain have serious and, in some cases, highly addictive and potentially deadly side effects. They must be considered as potential treatment options with great caution.

If we group natural supplements for chronic pain based on the level of scientific evidence of effectiveness we have three groups. Group A is PEA, and combination treatments with PEA are discussed above. In Group B are three supplements that currently have limited scientific research but show some promise and may emerge as future treatments in combination with PEA or stand-alone. These include Omega 3, GLA, and Honokiol. In Group C are vitamins and minerals that can help with some pain conditions, especially if you are deficient in one of these supplements. These include the B vitamins B1, B6, and B12, C, D3, and E. Minerals and plant extracts, including curcumin, ginger, melatonin, MSM, capsaicin, NAC, and saffron. There is scientific research to indicate that all of these supplements have some benefit in treating some forms of pain, but there is little or no evidence that they are effective individually or in combination in treating serious chronic pain. Melatonin, D3, E, and Omega 3 from food sources are part of the Prostatitis 360 Protocol. Finally, cannabis or CBD has been used by some men as a treatment for chronic prostatitis pain, but studies show the benefits to be minor to moderate at best, with potential side effects such as lower sperm count and sperm quality, which can impact male fertility. (7)

Conventional Medical Treatments for Chronic Prostatitis Pain

The following conventional medical treatments include treatments for severe chronic prostatitis pain. They include a wide range of pharmaceutical treatments as well as non-pharmaceutical treatments such as acupuncture and different versions of shock wave therapy.

Acupuncture

Acupuncture has gained widespread acceptance in the US as a scientifically proven and effective treatment for chronic prostatitis pain during the past 10 years. It is effective in treating pain but not the other symptoms of chronic prostatitis, such as urination symptoms, and it works for some but not all men with chronic prostatitis.

A 2023 meta-analysis of 17 studies, including RCT studies with 1,455 patients, reported significantly lower pain using both the CPSI and the VAS measures of pain. (5) Meta-analyses such as this that

CHAPTER 7
Chronic Pain Management

include RCT studies provide the strongest scientific validation of the effectiveness of medical treatments. Some individual studies have reported that it is typically effective in about 60% of patients and that the improvement in chronic pain ranges from 30% to approximately 50% when it works. Some studies have also looked at whether the benefits last beyond the initial treatment and confirmed effectiveness beyond the initial treatment period. A 2021 study of men with chronic prostatitis involved 20 sessions over 8 weeks and reported that 60.6% of the patients had a significant reduction in pain of at least 6 points on the CPSI pain scale. This study was particularly interesting because it included a 24-week follow-up to determine whether these pain reductions were lasting. The reduction in pain after 24 weeks remained stable. (6) A study of 100 patients with chronic prostatitis over a 24-week period reported a response rate of 92% and a 50% reduction in pain. (8) Acupuncture has clear benefits and clear limitations. It does not work for all men, and the benefits are limited to reducing pain by approximately 50%. It does not help with the other symptoms of chronic prostatitis. However, among conventional medical treatments, acupuncture has a very important advantage because there are no side effects. It is also relatively inexpensive, and in many cases, PPO and HMO health plans will pay for a basic course of treatment of 10 sessions over 8 to 10 weeks. This may not be adequate; many studies involve 20 sessions over 8 to 10 weeks. Many doctors specializing in pain medicine and pain clinics often include an acupuncturist on staff that focuses on treating pain as part of the practice. If you are part of a PPO, look for an in-network pain specialist or clinic that has an acupuncturist on staff. This may be the easiest way to get health insurance companies to approve and pay for acupuncture treatments.

Botox Prostate Injections

Research done during the past 15 years on the use of Botox to treat men with chronic prostatitis has been very promising, particularly in treating the pain symptoms of the condition. It has also been used with some success to treat BPH, IC/Painful Bladder Syndrome, and Overactive Bladder. A 2019 meta-analysis of Botox injections for chronic prostatitis involving six studies, including RCT studies and 283 patients, reported a significant decrease in pain as well as some improvements in urination symptoms in some of the studies. Most of the studies used 200 units of Botox injected into the prostate and tracked the outcomes for six months. (8)

A 2015 RCT study with 60 men included in the meta-analysis reported an impressive reduction in pain symptoms that remained consistent during the six-month follow-up period. In the study, 79.9% of the patients reported a 10-point or greater reduction in overall CPSI scores, and 82.1% of the patients reported an 8-point or greater reduction in pain on the VAS pain scale. (9) These results are very impressive both in terms of the extent of pain reduction and the higher percentage of patients who benefited. As a monotherapy, these results are comparable to studies of flower pollen, which saw Palmetto as a monotherapy treatment. There are, however, several issues with Botox that make it less attractive than flower pollen or saw palmetto as a treatment option. One of the studies in the meta-analysis tracked patient outcomes for 12 months and reported a drop off in pain reduction after 9 months. This means that the benefits of the treatment begin to fade after six months, and the treatment may need to be repeated every 9 to 12 months to be effective. A single 200-unit Botox injection course of treatment is very expensive, and the treatment becomes particularly expensive if it has to be repeated annually. Botox treatment for chronic prostatitis is not covered by health insurance. It may be difficult to find doctors with experience

CHAPTER 7
Chronic Pain Management

doing Botox injections for chronic prostatitis. Therefore, Botox injections as a treatment for chronic prostatitis may only be a viable option for men who can afford it and who have seen some benefit but have not attained a 50% or greater reduction in symptoms after implementing the complete Chronic Prostatitis 360 Protocol. Acupuncture and PEA, discussed above, may be much better treatment alternatives to try prior to considering Botox.

Shockwave Therapy

Shockwave therapy as a treatment for chronic prostatitis has been studied during the past 15 years but is not widely used in the US for chronic prostatitis. The two most common versions of shockwave therapy are called EWST and LIST. Meta-analyses done using both types of shock wave therapy report comparable benefits for chronic prostatitis patients. A 2021 study of 215 men with chronic prostatitis treated using EWST shockwave therapy and tracked for 12 months reported significant improvements. After 12 months, pain symptoms were reduced by 37.3%, urinary symptoms by 35.6%, quality of life improved by 53.6%, and the study reported significant improvement in ED symptoms. If we compare two so-called minimally invasive treatments, acupuncture and shockwave treatment, acupuncture is better at reducing pain, 50% vs. 37%, but acupuncture does not help with urinary and ED symptoms. On balance, shockwave therapy is the superior treatment for chronic prostatitis symptoms overall, except for individuals whose pain is the more severe symptom. In both cases, side effects, if any, are minor and rare. Shockwave therapy for chronic prostatitis requires special training and equipment. While it is available as a treatment for ED by private specialty clinics, it is not widely available as a treatment for chronic prostatitis. Most urologists do not offer shockwave therapy for ED or chronic prostatitis as part of their practice. Shockwave therapy is not covered by health insurance for either ED or chronic prostatitis. Shockwave therapy is, in short, a research or academic fact rather than a practical treatment option for most men with chronic prostatitis. PEA combined with saw palmetto or acupuncture are widely available and inexpensive treatment options for chronic prostatitis that offer better pain symptom reduction.

Pharmaceutical Treatments for Chronic Prostatitis Pain

Research done during the past 20 years has consistently shown that the traditional pharmaceutical drugs used to treat chronic prostatitis, including chronic prostatitis pain, are not effective. The most recent study is a 2022 meta-analysis of 25 studies involving a total of 3,514 patients that evaluated 26 of the most common individual and combination pharmaceutical treatments for chronic prostatitis. The study included the common prescription drugs used to treat chronic prostatitis, such as Tamsulosin and Levofloxacin, as well as a wide range of conventional chronic pain drugs, such as Doxazosin and Mepartricin that have been tested as potential treatments for chronic prostatitis. The study concluded that "there little is evidence" that traditional pharmaceutical drugs are effective in treating chronic prostatitis pain. (10) There are three drugs, however, that have proven in studies to be significantly better than placebo:

Daily 5mg Cialis: A Safe and Effective Conventional Drug Treatment

The only conventional medical drug treatment that has been proven to be safe and provide greater than 70% improvement in chronic prostatitis symptoms if used long term is daily 5mg Cialis in the

CHAPTER 7
Chronic Pain Management

PDE five class of drugs. Several recent studies using 5mg daily Cialis for a minimum of 3 months and normally requiring 6 months or more have proven effective in RCT studies.

Cialis Research

During the past five years, 7 RCT studies of 5mg Cialis have been conducted for treating chronic prostatitis. Many of these studies were short, lasting from 4 to 6 weeks. All the studies reported significant improvement in total CPSI scores and pain, urination, and quality of life scores. Unfortunately, there appear to have been no studies of 10, 15, or 20 milligrams of daily use of Cialis. A meta-analysis done by Alzahrani and colleagues in 2022 of seven RCT studies with 584 patients reported significant reductions in total CPSI scores as well as pain, urination, and quality of life scores. **(2)** A 6-week 2022 study by Tawfik and colleagues with 140 patients reported that 50.8% of the Cialis group had a 25% or greater reduction in total CPSI scores compared to just 5.4% for the placebo group. Urination and quality of life scores improved significantly, but the pain score remained unchanged in the Cialis group. **(3)** Another six-week study (Park, 2019) also reported improvements in all areas except the pain score. However, three-month studies (Pirola, 2020; Anas, 2023) report improvement in total CPSI scores, urination, quality of life, and pain scores. The 3-month 2023 Anas study reported that 79.6% of the patients had a substantial improvement in CPSI scores, including the pain score, as well as a substantial improvement in the ED score. **(4)** While the number of studies and the number of patients studied is limited, there are two preliminary conclusions we can draw from these studies. The first is that 5mg Cialis can provide significant improvement in chronic prostatitis symptoms, including pain symptoms if taken for three or more months. The second is that Cialis has the advantage of improving both chronic prostatitis and erectile dysfunction (ED) symptoms.

There is one long-term study, however, that suggests that Cialis can provide substantial improvement if taken for over a year. A 2019 study by Pinault and colleagues involved 25 patients who took Cialis for 15 months. The results in this study were very impressive, with 19 or 76% of the patients reporting a significant improvement or better, including 11 with substantial improvements and 7 with dramatic improvements, which came close to providing a cure for some of the seven patients. **(5)** Unfortunately, this is just one study with only 25 patients. If, in the future, there are more studies involving a larger number of patients, Cialis could emerge as a treatment comparable to saw palmetto or perhaps even flower pollen if you take it for longer than 6 months. There is one study that compared Cialis and flower pollen. The three-month study by Matsukawa and colleagues done in 2020 with 100 patients compared Cialis and Cernilton flower pollen. While both groups reported improvement, the pollen extract group reported that 50% of the patients had a 50% or greater improvement in their symptoms compared to just 8.9% for the Cialis group. **(6)** It is important to note that, unlike the five main chronic prostatitis phytotherapy, Cialis requires 6 to 9 months or more to see the full benefit. It has the important advantage of helping with erectile dysfunction. Therefore, adding Cialis to the five core phytotherapies may be a good strategy for men with ED. However, even if you do not have ED, Cialis may complement your phytotherapy treatment program because researchers believe that it improves the symptoms of chronic prostatitis in ways that are different from the five phytotherapies. The key difference between Cialis and the phytotherapies is that Cialis is a drug with greater potential for side effects. Studies show

CHAPTER 7
Chronic Pain Management

that side effects are rare and minor in most cases, but there is the potential for more serious side effects. It is important to carefully monitor Cialis for side effects, especially if you use it long-term. The side effects of Cialis are minor compared to other major prescription drugs used to treat chronic prostatitis, all of which have potentially serious side effects and are often discontinued by patients due to their side effects. Cialis is the only prescription drug that has been proven to be safe and effective in significantly reducing the symptoms of chronic prostatitis if taken for one year or more.

Despite the fact that Cialis is the only safe and effective prescription drug for chronic prostatitis, most urologists in the US are not familiar with Cialis as a treatment for chronic prostatitis and do not prescribe it. None of the 6 urologists I saw discussed much less prescribed Cialis as a treatment for chronic prostatitis. The best option may be to simply ask your primary care doctor for a prescription for Cialis. It is important to keep in mind that Cialis is a long-term treatment. It may take three months to see significant benefits, especially in your pain symptoms, and it may take 6 to 12 months or more before you see the full benefit of Cialis.

The five primary supplements recommended in the Prostatitis 360 Protocol have much more extensive scientific research, begin to work faster and achieve better overall results than Cialis. Nevertheless, I believe Cialis can complement the treatment options for men with chronic prostatitis. Cialis is part of the chronic Prostatitis 360 Protocol as an add-on treatment to the five primary supplements for chronic prostatitis for all men, especially for men with erectile dysfunction. I discuss Cialis in additional detail as a treatment for ED in chapter 9, which is dedicated to sexual health for men with chronic prostatitis.

Doxazosin

Doxazosin is a new "next generation" alpha-blocker that, in studies, has been reported to be more effective than a placebo stand-alone and particularly effective in combination with other drugs. Doxazosin combined with Duloxetine, a muscle relaxer, is the most promising of these combinations. A 2017 RCT study of 150 patients with chronic prostatitis was divided into groups; they compared 4 mg of Doxazosin to 4 mg of Doxazosin plus 60 mg of Duloxetine. Results were analyzed after 1, 3, and 6 months. After six months, 88.64% of the combination group reported a 25% improvement compared to just 56.10% for the Doxazosin-only group. The improvement after one month was relatively minor, while the improvement after three and six months was very similar. In other words, it takes approximately three months to see the full benefit of this combination treatment. There are, however, significant drawbacks to this drug. Studies show that up to 9.7% of patients have side effects. The most common side effects reported were headache and dizziness. (11)

Mepartricin

Mepartricin has been used for over 20 years to treat BPH and bladder problems. Several small RCT studies have reported that it is also effective in treating chronic prostatitis pain but not urination symptoms. A 2010 60-day study using 80 milligrams of Mepartricin reported an overall improvement of 70% and a 75% improvement in pain symptoms. There was no significant improvement in urinary symptoms. Side effects were few and minor. An earlier study by the same lead researcher using 40 milligrams for 60 days reported an overall improvement of 60% and a 63% improvement in pain symptoms. (12) More research is needed on both Mepartricin and the Doxazosin / Duloxetine combination. While the results of

CHAPTER 7
Chronic Pain Management

studies on these two drugs are impressive, they are not comparable in terms of the level of improvement and the number of studies done on flower pollen extract and saw palmetto and side effects remain a significant concern.

Chronic Pain Management Drugs

More recently, preliminary research has focused on four drugs used for chronic pain as potential emerging treatments for chronic prostatitis pain. Some of these drugs are promising:

Gabapentin

Gabapentin (Neurontin) and Pregabalin (Lyrica) are two common anti-epileptic drugs that have been tested as potential treatments for chronic prostatitis, with Gabapentin emerging in small preliminary studies as a potential treatment option for chronic prostatitis pain. A 2017 study involving 119 men with chronic prostatitis compared Gabapentin to Pregabalin during a 12-month period. After 12 months, 75% of the Gabapentin group reported at least a 50% reduction in pain compared to only 40% of the Pregabalin group. (13) More research is necessary, but this initial study is promising. While all prescription drugs have potential side effects and should be monitored carefully, Gabapentin is generally considered safe.

Amitriptyline

Most of the research on Amitriptyline has been done on the treatment of IC and Painful Bladder Syndrome (PBS) with a focus on pain and urination symptoms. The only data on the use of Amitriptyline for chronic prostatitis involves individual case studies that report some significant success with pain and urination symptoms. Several small studies have reported significant success in treating both the pain and urination symptoms of IC/PBS. (14) There is, however, a great deal of concern and many questions about the side effects of this drug, including potentially very serious side effects. Until there is clear, compelling scientific research on the use of Amitriptyline for chronic prostatitis, Gabapentin is a better drug alternative. And overall, acupuncture, Botox, and PEA are more effective treatment options.

Memantine

A Small number of limited studies of Memantine have reported significant improvements in chronic prostatitis pain symptoms. A 2009 RCT study evaluated 170 men with chronic prostatitis who took 20 mg/day of Memantine for six months. In the study 77% of the man in the Memantine group reported a significant improvement in pain and quality of life compared to only 16% for the men in the placebo group. There was, however, no improvement in urination symptoms. Side effects were minimal and included dizziness (7%), headache (5%) and tiredness (1%). If additional research confirms these results, Memantine may be a good option for treating the pain symptoms of chronic prostatitis. Until then, Gabapentin is a better option in terms of treating pain and has the added benefit of also treating urination symptoms. (15)

Gabapentin and the Doxazosin / Duloxetine combination stand out as the two best pharmaceutical pain drug treatments for chronic prostatitis pain based on the quality of the available research, overall effectiveness, and potential for side effects. In working with the plain specialist, these two drugs, along with acupuncture and Botox injections, should be the main focus of developing an individualized treatment plan. Most pain specialists will not be familiar with the best treatments for chronic prostatitis pain. This chapter will guide

CHAPTER 7
Chronic Pain Management

you in developing a successful working relationship with your pain specialist. The following is the best order in which to try these 6 treatments based on effectiveness, side effects, and cost:

1. PEA
2. Acupuncture
3. Botox
4. 5mg Cialis
5. Doxazosin / Duloxetine combination
6. Gabapentin

Where to Start

Prior to working with a pain specialist, the best place to start is with the combination of PEA/Polydatin and Saw Palmetto, which are safe, effective, and inexpensive chronic prostatitis pain treatments that don't require a prescription. The best traditional medical treatment for chronic prostatitis is 5 mg daily Cialis. Cialis treats the full range of chronic prostatitis symptoms, including pain. In terms of traditional medical treatments, you can work with your primary care doctor for a Cialis prescription.

CHAPTER 8
Chronic Prostatitis Urination Symptoms

This chapter is for men needing additional help improving their urination symptoms. Urination problems are the second most common symptom for men with chronic prostatitis. For many men, urination symptoms go hand in hand with pain, the most common symptom of chronic prostatitis, and there is a more or less consistent improvement in both symptoms after implementing the Prostatitis 360 Protocol. This chapter is for men who have seen significant improvement in both pain and urination symptoms after implementing the chronic Prostatitis 360 Protocol but for whom the improvement in urination symptoms has significantly lagged the improvement in pain symptoms. In other words, this chapter is for men needing additional help improving their urination symptoms. The focus of this chapter, therefore, is on additional treatment measures that can be taken to improve the urination symptoms of chronic prostatitis.

CHAPTER 8
Chronic Prostatitis Urination Symptoms

Lifestyle

Lifestyle changes can play an important role in improving urination symptoms. Many of the lifestyle changes the target urination symptoms focus on some aspect of bladder health, which is, in many cases, the primary underlying cause of many urination symptoms not directly caused by chronic prostatitis. While the Prostatitis 360 Protocol addresses many aspects of bladder health, there is a wide range of additional treatment options to improve bladder health.

Lifestyle Risk Factors

Studies show that obesity, smoking, and being over 60 are risk factors for Overactive Bladder or OAB. If you have chronic prostatitis and have these risk factors for OAB, your symptoms may be a combination of chronic prostatitis and OAB or borderline OAB. In this case, you may need to treat both conditions. In this chapter, we discuss treatments for OAB. Interstitial Cytosis, or IC, is another bladder-related condition with similar urination symptoms. However, IC primarily impacts women and is much less common among men. At the same time, these risk factors make it more likely to have OAB. If you have these risk factors, treating your urination symptoms starts with stopping smoking and managing your weight.

Diet

Diet may be the most important lifestyle change to improve urination symptoms. For men with chronic prostatitis and those with related bladder health conditions such as IC and OAB, the bladder becomes highly sensitive to acidic foods and drinks. Highly acidic foods irritate the bladder and urethra, which results in pain, bloating, and urination problems. In chronic prostatitis, acidic foods are a problem because they cause inflammation of the urethra and prostate. However, the same acidic foods are also a problem for some men because they irritate the bladder and urethra.

In most cases, inflammation and irritation go hand in hand, but for some men, the Prostatitis 360 Protocol is successful in addressing inflammation, but bladder and urethra irritation remains a problem. The primary issue with bladder irritation is the lining of the bladder wall and urethra. Acidic foods and foods high in histamine that trigger mass cell activation syndrome or MCAS are the greatest irritants of the bladder wall. There is a great deal of overlap between bladder health diets and the Chronic Prostatitis 360 Diet, but there are some important differences as well as differences in emphasis. The bladder health diet places a greater emphasis on acidic and irritating beverages. Appendix II lists bladder-irritating foods that should be eliminated and suggestions for acceptable substitutes.

Bladder Irritating Beverages:

1. Alcohol. All alcoholic drinks, including beer and wine.
2. Caffeine. All caffeine-based drinks, such as coffee, tea, and colas, including decaf, as well as foods with cocoa, such as chocolate, contain caffeine.
3. Carbonated drinks. All types, including soft drinks, seltzers, and carbonated mineral waters.
4. Citrus fruit juices
5. Tomatoes and tomato-based foods such as salsas, sauces, and juices.
6. Artificial sweeteners.

A 2016 study found that removing the beverages above and replacing them with water significantly lowered urination symptoms

CHAPTER 8
Chronic Prostatitis Urination Symptoms

after three weeks. (1) Studies also show that carbonated drinks are strongly associated with urination symptoms and rank just below alcohol and caffeine. If you have followed the Chronic Prostatitis 360 Diet and have eliminated alcohol and caffeine but not carbonated drinks, removing them from your diet may improve your urination symptoms.

There are some beverages that soothe or calm the bladder in addition to plain water.

Bladder Soothing Beverages:

1. Warm milk
2. Warm water
3. Peppermint tea
4. Chamomile tea

Studies show that peppermint tea soothes the lining of the bladder and calms small muscle bowel spasms. Peppermint tea may be a good replacement for coffee and green tea. It has a bolder taste and aroma compared to chamomile tea, which can be bland for coffee and green tea drinkers. Peppermint tea is not readily available, but you can find it online and at stores with a large specialty tea selection, such as Sprouts, which is found in many parts of the US.

Bladder Irritating Foods

The following foods cause the greatest irritation to the bladder and should be entirely removed from your diet. These dietary changes are part of the Prostatitis 360 Diet, but if you have not been careful following this diet and you continue to experience significant urination symptoms, removing these foods may help.

Spicy Foods: Chiles, wasabi, horseradish, vinegar, chili, hot peppers and MSG

Acidic Foods: Citrus fruits, including lemons, limes, oranges, and grapefruit. Tomatoes and tomato-based products.

Chocolate: All forms of chocolate, including milk, dark, and any food that includes chocolate. White chocolate and carob are fine and are good alternatives, but white chocolate should be eaten in moderation because of the high sugar content.

Salt: Salty foods and snacks. Replace salt with herbs in cooking. Small amounts of salt occasionally may be tolerated.

Cuisines: Mexican, Thai, and Indian.

Other: Some strict low acid / anti-inflammation diets also recommend removing sugar and dairy.

Healthy Bladder Foods

The following are the best foods to minimize urination symptoms. Most other vegetables, fish, and non-citrus low-acid fruits are fine, but these are the best.

Fruits: Blueberries, pears, bananas, honeydew melon and watermelon.

CHAPTER 8
Chronic Prostatitis Urination Symptoms

Vegetables: Broccoli, brussels sprouts, cauliflower, carrots, celery, cucumber, peas, mushrooms, squash, sweet potatoes, white potatoes, and zucchini.

Meat and protein: Chicken, turkey, pork, beef, and lamb. Eggs. Avoid highly processed meats that are usually high in salt, such as bacon, sandwich meats, and sausage.

Fish: Salmon, tuna, and scrimp.

Low Histamine Gluten-Free Diet

A low histamine gluten-free diet is part of the Chronic Prostatitis 360 anti-inflammation diet. If you have not followed that part of the diet, carefully remove all sources of gluten and histamine from your diet. Strictly following that part of the diet may improve your urination symptoms in 60 to 90 days. Histamine and histamine intolerance is a contributing factor to Interstitial Cystitis / Bladder Pain Syndrome (IC/PBS), a condition that primarily affects women. IC/PBS causes urination symptoms, but the defining symptom is bladder pain and bloating. Almost all the research on IC/PBS has been done with women. Therefore, we do not know how effective treatments for this condition are for the small percentage of men who have IC/PBS. If you have urination symptoms, have not responded well to the Prostatitis 360 Protocol, and also have painful bladder symptoms, implementing a strict low histamine gluten-free diet should, in most cases, improve both the bladder pain and urination symptoms if you have both urination and painful bladder symptoms. In that case, you may have IC/PBS as the primary cause or a secondary contributing factor to your symptoms, and you should work with a urologist who has experience treating the condition. There is a wide range of natural and alternative treatments as well as conventional medical treatments for IC/PBS. The IC Network at ic-network.com is a good place to start.

Supplements for Urination Symptoms

A wide range of nutraceuticals, including vitamins, supplements, and phytotherapies, have been scientifically proven in rigorous RCT studies to help with the symptoms of overactive bladder (OAB), a broad term used to describe a wide range of urination symptoms and problems.

A. The most common urination problems for men with chronic prostatitis are listed below. These are also the most common symptoms of OAB as a standalone medical condition, with one important exception. Pain and burning during urination set chronic prostatitis urination symptoms apart from the classic symptoms of OAB. Several other conditions, including pelvic floor dysfunction, BPH, and IC/PBS, overlap some of the symptoms of OAB listed below.

1. Frequency: Urinating (voiding is the medical term) more than six times during the day. Sometimes also a sensation that you still need to urinate after urinating
2. Urgency: The need to go is intense
3. Hesitancy: Difficulty starting a urine stream
4. Nocturia: Urinating more than once overnight during sleep
5. Incomplete emptying: post urination dribble
6. Weak stream: Low volume, slow and sometimes short urination
7. Chronic condition: the urination symptoms are chronic; they usually do not come and go

CHAPTER 8
Chronic Prostatitis Urination Symptoms

B. Other Urination Problems
1. Incontinence: Unintentional or involuntary "leaking" of urine and weak control of urination. Incontinence is, in turn, subdivided into stress and urge incontinence. Although it is believed to be more common among women, it happens to men as well. Incontinence typically starts after age 40 and increases with age thereafter. It is considered a separate medical condition.
2. Polyuria: frequent intense volume urination is less common and rarely a chronic condition
3. Bladder urine retention: not fully emptying the bladder does occur with OAB but is more common in men with BPH

Five Core Chronic Prostatitis Supplements

These five core supplements in the Prostatitis 360 Protocol are used to treat chronic prostatitis successfully in many cases because they treat both the pain and urination symptoms. Since these are the two dominant symptoms of chronic prostatitis, a successful treatment must address both. Rigorous scientific research done during the past 25 years has consistently shown that all five are effective in treating not only the pain but also the urination symptoms of chronic prostatitis in most cases. Saw palmetto and flower pollen, in particular, have been extensively studied and widely used to treat the urination symptoms of chronic prostatitis, BPH, and overactive bladder. However, as always, individual results vary, and the level of effectiveness in treating urination symptoms will vary. If you have been taking all five for more than 6 months and have seen substantial improvement in your pain symptoms but less improvement in your urination symptoms, it may mean that your urination symptoms are more persistent and slower to respond to the Prostatitis 360 Protocol. You may need additional treatments for your chronic urination symptoms. There are several supplements that have been proven to complement the five primary chronic prostatitis supplements when they are combined to improve urination symptoms further. There are also standalone supplements that have been proven to improve urination symptoms. There is so much overlap between the urination symptoms of chronic prostatitis and those of OAB and BPH that many of the supplements used for OAB and BPH are also used to treat the urination symptoms of chronic prostatitis.

Overactive Bladder / OAB

The urination symptoms of chronic prostatitis mimic so many of the urination symptoms of OAB that it's important to understand how the two conditions are different to rule out the possibility that you have both conditions. This is especially true because 50% of men with chronic prostatitis are over 50 because OAB is increasingly more common after age 50. There is also, in other words, an age overlap between the two conditions. However, important differences between chronic prostatitis and OAB can help you distinguish between the two conditions. OAB is a bladder condition. The urination system symptoms are typically accompanied by moderate to severe bladder symptoms, including bladder spasms, cramping, and burning pain in the bladder. Some men with chronic prostatitis do experience some bladder symptoms, such as cramping, but they are typically mild.

CHAPTER 8
Chronic Prostatitis Urination Symptoms

Enlarged Prostate / BPH

The urination symptoms of chronic prostatitis also overlap a great deal with the urination symptoms of BPH. There is also a significant age overlap because 50% of men with chronic prostatitis are over 50, and BPH is a medical condition that predominantly impacts men over 50 and is more common as men age after 50. However, as we discussed in Chapter 1, it is relatively easy to distinguish between chronic prostatitis and BPH with an ultrasound to measure the size of the prostate. For men over 50 with chronic prostatitis, BPH is so common in men over 50 that it is possible to have both conditions. If you are over 50 and you currently do not have BPH, it is important to continuously monitor your prostate size because BPH is very common among men over 50 and is increasingly more common as you age. The prostate ultrasound is an easy, simple, and inexpensive test. There are no guidelines for how often this test should be repeated after age 50, but a good rule of thumb is to do it every five years.

Saw Palmetto Combinations

Individual studies and meta-analyses done during the past 25 years show that saw palmetto extract (SPE) is effective as a standalone treatment for urination symptoms in many cases. If, however, you have already been taking Saw Palmetto along with flower pollen and quercetin as part of the 360 Protocol for at least six months and still need additional help with your urination symptoms, there are Saw Palmetto combinations that have proven to be effective.

Nettle Root Extract

Nettle Root Extract (NRE), also known as Stinging Nettle Root, has been widely used in Europe for over 20 years to treat BPH and chronic prostatitis. In Europe, it's manufactured by pharmaceutical companies, and all the studies discussed below are based on the

NRE made by pharmaceutical companies. NRE, as a standalone treatment, has been shown to be effective in treating urination symptoms in several studies.

A particularly interesting 6-month double-blind placebo-controlled RCT study done in 2005 by Safarinejad and colleagues with 588 patients who took 500 mg of NRE reported significant improvement in 81% of the patients in the NRE group compared to 16% for the placebo group. As measured by IPSS, the International Prostate Symptom Score, overall urination symptoms improved by 40% for the NRE group compared to just 7% for the placebo group. The peak flow rate improved by 8.2 mL/s for the NRE group compared to 3.4 mL/s for the placebo group. This is a significant improvement for the NRE group. The peak flow rate for men typically ranges from 10 to 20 mL/s. A peak flow rate of 15 m/Ls is considered normal. The peak flow rate is a measure of the strength or weakness of urine flow. A weak urine stream is a common symptom of urination problems. A follow-up done 18 months after the study showed that the improvements achieved in the study remained in place for those men who continued treatment with NRE, and most men chose to continue the treatment. None of the men in the study reported any significant side effects. (2)

However, most of the high-quality studies with NRE have combined NRE and SPE. A 2019 study by Kirschner-Hermann and colleagues compared the combination of SPE and NRE to two commonly used prescription drugs, Finasteride and Tamsulosin. The study used 160 mg of SPE and 120 milligrams of NRE taken twice a day. The SPE & NRE combination was significantly better than the placebo in treating urination symptoms with no side effects reported and comparable to Finasteride and Tamsulosin, both of which have serious potential side effects and are often discontinued

CHAPTER 8
Chronic Prostatitis Urination Symptoms

due to side effects the patients can't tolerate, especially after long-term use. (3)

Nocturia, waking up two or more times to urinate during sleep, is a particularly problematic urination symptom for men with chronic prostatitis. The poor sleep caused by nocturia is believed to negatively impact immune health, gut health, and depression, which in turn directly or indirectly negatively impact chronic prostatitis symptoms. Studies show that the combination of SPE and NRE can improve nocturia symptoms. The study done by Oelke and colleagues in 2014 with 922 patients who took one 120 mg NRE and 160 mg of SPE twice a day for 24 weeks saw a 50% improvement versus placebo in their nocturia symptoms with nighttime urination declining from an average of 2.1 to 1 per night. The study also compared the NRE and SPE combination with the commonly used drugs Finasteride and Tamsulosin and reported comparable results without the potentially serious side effects of those two drugs. (4)

A common objection to nutraceuticals like SPE and an NRE is that, in some cases, there is a lack of long-term studies to determine how effective they are after 6 or 12 months. However, there are long-term studies in the case of SPE and NRE. A long-term study by Lopatkin and colleagues, published in 2007, involved 257 men who took 120 milligrams of NRE and 160 milligrams of SPE twice a day for 96 weeks. After 24 weeks, the researchers reported 53% lower IPSS scores, a 19% improvement in peak urinary flow, and a 44% decrease in residual urine volume in the bladder. These improvements were significantly better than placebo after 24 weeks. The improvements held steady after 48 weeks and 96 weeks.

There is, in short, compelling scientific evidence that adding nettle root extract to the Prostatitis 360 phytotherapy treatment protocol that includes Saw Palmetto can significantly improve most urination symptoms. The typical dosage used in studies in Europe has been 120 milligrams taken twice a day. In the US, NRE is sold in much higher doses. The NOW brand sells a 250 mg version, and Swanson has a 500 mg version of NRE, both of which are good options. Most other US brands sell NRE with 1,000 mg or more. In my case, I take the Swanson 500 mg version once a day, and it has been very effective. There is no evidence that these higher doses are effective, and there was no research about the safety of taking high-dose NRE in the long term. It is generally not a good idea to take high doses of any supplement unless it is supported by scientific evidence and has been studied long-term for side effects.

Pumpkin Seed Oil

Pumpkin seed oil (PSO) is believed to be effective in reducing urinary symptoms in part by helping to relax the bladder, decrease the sense of urinary urgency, decrease bladder spasms, and increase bladder capacity. Several rigorous scientific studies done during the past 25 years have reported that pumpkin seed oil (PSO) can significantly improve urination symptoms and quality of life. The level of improvement reported in these studies ranges from a 30% to 46% improvement in urinary symptoms and quality of life. Studies show that NRE is more effective than PSO, but how you respond to each will vary. You may find that PSO is more effective in your case. If NRE does not work for you, PSO is another option. As a standalone treatment, PSO is not a cure for these symptoms, nor will it provide a dramatic improvement. A moderate improvement in your urinary symptoms and quality of life can nevertheless have a significant overall impact. If you have seen, for example, a 50% improvement in your urination symptoms by implementing the Prostatitis 360 Protocol, an additional 20% improvement, for example, achieved by adding PSO, can make a significant difference in your symptoms and quality of life. This

CHAPTER 8
Chronic Prostatitis Urination Symptoms

scenario is just a theoretical example. Your situation and the results you achieve by adding PSO, NRE, and the other nutraceuticals I discussed below will vary.

A study done in 2000 by Friederich and colleagues with 2,245 patients who took 1,000 mg of pumpkin seed oil reported significant improvements after 12 weeks. There was an average 41% reduction in urination symptoms and a 46% improvement in quality of life. Side effects were rare and minor, with 96% of the participants reporting no side effects and 4% reporting minor side effects. (5)

A limited number of studies of nutraceuticals, such as pumpkin seed oil, focus on OAB. The 2014 study by Nishimura and colleagues focused on OAB symptoms not related to conditions such as BPH and used the OAB symptom scale or OABSS to analyze the results. In the study, 45 patients took 10,000 mg of PSO for 12 weeks. After 12 weeks, the overall OABSS declined by 4.4 points for the PSO group compared to 2.7 points for the placebo group. The PSO group achieved an overall OABSS reduction of 38%, a 42% reduction in daytime frequency, a 31% reduction in nocturia, and a 93% reduction in urgency. There are, however, two limitations to this study. The dosage used is 10 times higher than most studies of PSO. Most studies use 1,000 mg, and this study used 10,000 mg. The other difference is the variety of pumpkin seed oil used in this study. Most studies in the US and Europe use various PSOs known by the scientific name *Cucurbita Pepo*. This study used a variety of PSO commonly harvested in Asia, which is known by the scientific name *Cucurbita Maxima*. This study did not report any significant side effects after 12 weeks, but there is no data on the long-term side effects of taking such a large dose of PSO. We also do not know if the difference in the variety of PSO used significantly impacted the results reported in the study. (6) Another study that focused on OAB used the combination of 87.5% PSO and

12.5% equol a soy extract. In this study by Shim and colleagues done in 2014, 120 participants took the PSO soy extract combination for 12 weeks. The researchers used six different symptom measures from the OABSS, including urination frequency, urgency, incontinence frequency, maximum urgency score, nocturia, and the overall OAB symptom score, and reported significant improvements in all six measures of the OAB symptom scale. (7) A 2017 study by Leibbrand and colleagues involved 60 men who took 500 milligrams of PSO for three months. The researchers reported a 30% reduction in total IPSS scores, significant reductions in nocturia, and a significant improvement in the quality-of-life score. (8)

In 2016, Damiano and colleagues analyzed 6 RCT studies of PSO used for urinary symptoms, including four studies that reported quality-of-life results. The researchers reported that all six studies showed significant improvements in urinary symptoms. The four studies that included quality of life scores also reported significant improvements in quality of life. (9)

Most studies of PSO have used a 1,000 mg to 1,500 mg dosage per day. Three established, widely available brands in the US, NOW, Swanson, and Puritan Pride, sell 1,000 mg of PSO. You can experiment with increasing the daily dose to 2,000 to determine if it's more effective.

Lycopene

Lycopene using a dose of 25 mg is part of the chronic prostatitis 360 protocol to enhance the effectiveness of saw palmetto. There is research that doses ranging from 8mg to 1,000 mg per day are effective in significantly improving urination symptoms. The 2019 study by Li and colleagues used 127 patients with moderate to severe LUTS. The patients took 500 milligrams of lycopene two

CHAPTER 8
Chronic Prostatitis Urination Symptoms

times a day for 16 weeks. The researchers reported that IPSS, quality of life, and QMAX all significantly improved after 16 weeks. (10) QMAX is a measure of the maximum urine flow rate or a way to measure the strength of urine flow. Two comprehensive reviews, one done by Cicero in 2019 and another by Kutwin in 2022, analyzed studies of a total of over 1,000 patients with moderate to severe LUTS. The patients took 10 milligrams to 500 milligrams of lycopene twice a day from two weeks to six months. Most of the patients reported significant improvements in most categories of urination symptoms. (11) (12) A very interesting small study done in 2022 by Carrasco and colleagues compared 10 healthy men to 10 men with moderate BPH. In the study, both groups used extra virgin olive oil enriched with 8 milligrams of lycopene for 30 days. IPSS and nocturia improved significantly, sleep quality also improved, and the level of C-reactive protein significantly declined. C-reactive protein is a commonly used indicator of inflammation in the body. (13)

It is important to note that all the studies use lycopene in supplement form. While tomatoes are a rich food source of lycopene, they are also highly acidic and should generally be avoided on the prostatitis 360 anti-inflammation diet. You do not have to eat tomatoes and tomato-based products to take advantage of the benefits of lycopene.

There is substantial scientific evidence that lycopene can significantly improve urination symptoms. If you have been taking 25 milligrams of lycopene as part of the phytotherapy component of the prostatitis 360 protocol for three months or more and you still need additional help with urination symptoms, lycopene is another option if NRE and PSO are not effective. Studies have safely used up to 500 milligrams taken twice a day. In the US lycopene is generally not sold in higher doses above 40mg. Puritan Pride and

Carlyle have established brands offering 40 mg of lycopene. I use the 21st-century brand of 25-milligram lycopene. If you are currently taking 25 milligrams of lycopene as part of the protocol, you can increase your dose to 25 milligrams three times a day or take 40 milligrams twice a day from Puritan Pride or Carlyle to triple your dose of lycopene.

Pygeum Africanum

Pygeum Africanum comes from the bark of the African plum tree. Urologists sold and prescribed it throughout western, central, and Eastern Europe under the brand name Tadenan. It was introduced in 1992 by Viatris, a leading European pharmaceutical company, and discontinued in 2022 due to concerns about the environmental impact and sustainability of harvesting the bark. It is still widely available in the US as an over-the-counter supplement sold by several leading supplement manufacturers. It is unclear what the long-term future is for Pygeum Africanum. It was extensively studied in the 1990s as a treatment for the urination symptoms of BPH. Several studies and meta-analyses reported modest but significant improvements in nocturia, residual urine volume, and overall urination symptoms. A meta-analysis by Wilt and colleagues 2002 analyzed 18 studies with 1,562 participants done between 1996 in 2000. Most of the studies used 100 milligrams of Pygeum Africanum, and the study periods ranged from 30 to 122 days. Most of the patients in the Pygeum Africanum groups improved twice as much as in the placebo groups. There was an average 19% decline in nocturia and a 24% decline and residual urine volume. (14) Unfortunately, most of this research was done using the Tadenan product, which is no longer sold in Europe and has never been available in the US. There is very little rigorous research that is more recent and that has not used Tadenan.

CHAPTER 8
Chronic Prostatitis Urination Symptoms

Despite its many limitations, I believe that Pygeum Africanum can be a valid option if, after 6 months of taking pumpkin seed, nettle root extract, or lycopene, they are not effective. Studies show that pumpkin seed oil, nettle root extract, and lycopene are more effective, but your experience may differ. Studies also show that side effects are rare, minor, and inexpensive. So, there is little risk in experimenting with the product. If you're taking any prescription drugs, of course, as always, you should research potential drug interactions and discuss them with your doctor. The typical dosage studied is 100 mg. Solaray is an established brand that sells 100 mg and 50mg versions of Pygeum in the US.

Equol, Green Tea and Beta-Sitosterol

There was some limited emerging research on using equol, derived from soy and green tea, to treat urination symptoms. Beta-sitosterol is available standalone and is also found in saw palmetto, pumpkin seed oil, and *Pygeum Africanum*. It has been studied in the past as a treatment for urination symptoms, but the research is very limited. There is promising emerging research on Equol and green tea and some established research on beta-sitosterol, but the research is too limited and it is too early to seriously consider them as treatment options. If additional substantial research emerges in the future that confirms their effectiveness, they may deserve serious consideration.

Conventional Medicine for OAB, BPH, and IC/PBS

This chapter's diet, lifestyle, and supplements are intended to address the urination symptoms of men with chronic prostatitis. If you suspect you have OAB, BPH, or IC/PBS, you should work with your urologist to diagnose the condition and develop a treatment program. The diet, lifestyle, and supplements discussed in this chapter are not alternatives to working with a urologist if you are diagnosed with OAB, PBH, or IC/PBS, but they can complement the conventional medical treatment provided by your urologist. It's important to note that, unlike conventional medical treatment for chronic prostatitis, conventional medical treatment for OAB, PBH, and IC/PBS is generally more successful. However, as always, you must be careful with the potential short-term and long-term side effects of using prescription drugs. If you are diagnosed with OAB or BPH and you find that prescription drug treatments involve serious or unacceptable side effects, the supplements discussed above can be a potential alternative. They may also allow you to significantly reduce the dosage of the prescription drug by adding a supplement that successfully complements the drug and lowers or eliminates the side effects. If you're currently taking any prescription drugs, as always, you should discuss the use of any supplements with your doctor prior to starting the use of any supplements. If, on the other hand, you have been forced to discontinue a prescription drug treatment due to serious side effects, the supplements discussed above can be potential alternatives. Your doctor may discourage you from trying some of these supplements because many doctors in the US have a strong bias against supplements in general, and many are not familiar with the scientifically proven benefits of certain supplements. The supplements discussed above have a good safety record compared to prescription drugs with rare and minor side effects in every study cited above. If you are taking prescription drugs, you should, of course, discuss potential drug interactions with your doctor, but I also think you should do your own research about potential drug interactions. Once again, your doctors may discourage you from taking supplements because of a general bias against supplements on the part of many doctors, even when there are no known drug interactions.

CHAPTER 9
Erectile Dysfunction and Chronic Prostatitis

Sexual side effects are the third most common category of symptoms impacting most men with chronic prostatitis, following pain and urination symptoms. Sexual side effects include erectile dysfunction, premature ejaculation, and painful ejaculation in approximately that order. Painful ejaculation is more common among men with chronic pelvic floor pain. Erectile dysfunction is approximately three times more common among men with chronic prostatitis compared to the general population. In the general population of men between 20 and 70, approximately 22% have some form of erectile dysfunction compared to 62% for men with chronic prostatitis and chronic pelvic floor pain. The prevalence of erectile dysfunction begins to converge between the general population and men with chronic prostatitis after age 50, when it reaches 50% for the general population and 67% for men with chronic prostatitis. By age 70, it is 75% and 87%, respectively. (1) (2). The reason for this disparity between men with chronic prostatitis and men in the general population is not understood.

However, unlike the pain and urination symptoms of chronic prostatitis, the causes of erectile dysfunction are better understood, and the treatment options are more practical for most men, including men with chronic prostatitis.

Many men with erectile dysfunction have underlying conditions that cause or contribute to their symptoms, including diabetes, heart disease, hypertension, and BPH. The most effective approach to treating erectile dysfunction for these men is to treat the underlying condition. When the underlying condition is treated, the erectile treatments are significantly more effective. If you treat the underlying condition, you are less likely to require higher-dose ED drugs, which are associated with more and more serious side effects. While serious side effects are rare, they do occur, especially in men with underlying conditions such as heart disease, and can be very serious, including blindness and death. The FDA reported, for example, 128 deaths in a 7.5-month period in 2001 for men taking Viagra. (3) One analysis reported 50 deaths per one million prescriptions of Viagra, usually involving men with heart disease. (4)

Strategy for the Use of ED Drugs

The best strategy for men who need to take ED drugs, especially if they have an underlying condition such as heart disease, hypertension, or chronic prostatitis, is first to treat or control the underlying condition. Make lifestyle and diet changes that will enhance the effectiveness of ED drugs. Take the lowest dose necessary for effectiveness. Choose Tadalafil versus Viagra if Tadalafil is effective. The ideal strategy is to treat or control the underlying condition, implement diet and lifestyle changes, and use 5 mg daily Tadalafil (brand name Cialis), which has few and minor,

CHAPTER 9
Erectile Dysfunction and Chronic Prostatitis

if any, side effects if it is effective. In fact, as we will discuss below, 5 mg daily Tadalafil is effective for many men with ED, including men with more serious ED and underlying conditions such as heart disease or chronic prostatitis. On the other hand, if you don't treat or control the underlying condition and don't implement the diet and lifestyle changes discussed below, you may become dependent on higher doses of ED drugs, which involve more serious side effects.

Medical Care: Doctors & Tests

It is important to work with your primary doctor and urologist to understand and manage your ED. ED is often an indicator of underlying health problems that routine medical testing often does not detect. Some early-stage underlying conditions, such as prediabetes and prehypertension, may be overlooked in routine testing as being within normal range. Direct causes of ED, such as low testosterone and low free testosterone, are not routinely tested. You need to work with your primary care doctor and any other specialists to do a battery of tests to rule out common underlying conditions that cause or contribute to ED and direct causes of ED, such as low free testosterone. A basic battery of tests should include:

Physical exam. This should include careful examination of your penis and testicles and checking your nerves for sensation.

Blood tests. The blood test should include tests for heart disease, diabetes (including prediabetes), hypertension / pre-hypertension, total and free testosterone, thyroid function, estradiol, DHEA, homocysteine, and SHGB levels. It is important to test for free testosterone rather than total testosterone alone. It is free testosterone that impacts ED. You can have normal or even high total testosterone, but if free testosterone is low, you are likely to have ED. If free testosterone is low, it is important to test for SHGB, which regulates the level of free testosterone. Therefore, if you have ED, it is best to test the level of SHGB in the initial blood test. I discuss the supplements below to lower the level of SHGB. High levels of estradiol can decrease levels of testosterone. I also discuss the supplements below to decrease estradiol levels. Low DHEA can lower testosterone levels. I also discuss how to supplement with DHEA and homocysteine.

Urine tests (urinalysis). Like blood tests, urine tests are used to look for signs of diabetes and other underlying health conditions.

Ultrasound. An ultrasound of the penis is used to determine if the flow of blood to and from the penis is normal or if there are blood flow problems. This test can identify local causes of blood flow problems and signs of heart disease or diabetes.

Psychological exam. Your doctor should ask questions to screen for depression, severe anxiety, and other possible psychological causes of erectile dysfunction.

This is the battery of tests that should be done in your initial consultation with your primary care doctor and your urologist. Unfortunately, the reality is that in many cases, your doctor will prescribe a high dose of Viagra or Cialis after asking a few basic questions about your health and checking your health history and then schedule a follow-up appointment to see how those drugs work. This is very common, especially in HMO settings in the context of a typical 15-minute HMO appointment with your doctor. It is up to you as the patient to insist on having these tests and exams performed to understand and properly treat your condition, including any underlying causes of your ED. Even though testing

CHAPTER 9
Erectile Dysfunction and Chronic Prostatitis

for free testosterone is very important, many HMOs, including the largest HMO in the US, do not have a code in their system for ordering a free testosterone test as part of a blood test. In other words, the doctor cannot order a free testosterone test. You can insist on some kind of manual override of the system or simply incur the expense of having this test done at an independent lab.

If initial testing finds possible underlying causes or risk factors for your ED, such as hypertension/prehypertension or diabetes/prediabetes, it's important to treat these underlying conditions while starting the use of ED medications and supplements. You may need to start with a higher dose of Viagra, for example, 50, 75, or 100 mg, but the goal should be to treat the underlying conditions and use the lowest dose necessary for effectively treating your ED. Ideally, you reach the point where 5 mg daily of Cialis is enough to treat your ED. Unlike higher doses of Viagra, Cialis, and other ED medications, which can have serious, even very serious, side effects, 5 mg daily Cialis has proven in extensive testing to be effective and has few, if any, minor side effects. In addition to treating or controlling underlying conditions, a combination of supplements, diet, and lifestyle changes can help many men achieve the goal of relying on 5 milligrams of daily Cialis as their primary ED prescription drug treatment. Some men, especially men under the age of 40 or 45, may be able to resolve their ED condition with the combination of treating underlying conditions, supplements, and diet and lifestyle changes alone, but realistically for many men, especially men over 50, where age is a contributing factor, the goal should be to use the lowest possible dose of ED medication. You should work with your doctors to treat and manage underlying conditions. In the sections below, we discuss the use of supplements, diet, and lifestyle changes such as regular aerobic exercise. We also discuss the use of 5 milligrams of

Cialis alone and in combination with supplements and other ED medications.

Peripheral Neuropathy & ED

There is a consensus in the medical community based on decades of extensive medical research about physical inactivity, obesity, hypertension, metabolic syndrome, and/or cardiovascular diseases as underlying health conditions that cause or lead to ED. Metabolic syndrome is a condition that includes a combination of risk factors specific to cardiovascular disease. These include abdominal obesity, high blood pressure, impaired fasting glucose, high triglyceride levels, and low HDL cholesterol levels. If you have one or a combination of these conditions, we have discussed above the importance of working with your doctors to treat these conditions as part of the overall treatment plan for your erectile dysfunction.

The role of peripheral neuropathy as another major underlying health condition that causes or leads to ED is not widely discussed in the medical community in the US. However, recent research clearly shows a strong association between peripheral neuropathy and ED. A study of men over 40 in the US done by Hicks and colleagues in 2021 demonstrated a strong association between peripheral neuropathy and ED. The authors concluded that "We found a robust association of erectile dysfunction with peripheral neuropathy in US men ≥40 years of age. This association was pronounced in the absence of diabetes and persisted after adjusting for traditional risk factors." (11) If you have peripheral neuropathy, there is a strong likelihood that it is related to your erectile dysfunction. In other words, even if you do not have any other risk factors or underlying conditions, if you have peripheral neuropathy, it may explain why you have ED. As in the case of the other risk factors and underlying causes, it is important to work with your

CHAPTER 9
Erectile Dysfunction and Chronic Prostatitis

doctors to treat and manage your peripheral neuropathy as part of an overall plan to treat your ED.

Unfortunately, the treatment of peripheral neuropathy is in many ways very similar to the treatment of chronic prostatitis in the US. While the success rate of traditional medical treatment for peripheral neuropathy is better than chronic prostatitis, the overall success rate is low compared to many other conditions. Traditional medical treatment places a great deal of emphasis on pharmaceutical drugs. It largely ignores natural alternative treatments such as supplements, even though supplements, for example, have proven to be effective in rigorous scientific research for many individuals with peripheral neuropathy. Here, as in the case of chronic prostatitis, it's up to you, the patient, to take greater direct personal responsibility for managing the condition and identify proven alternative treatment options for this condition in addition to working with your doctors. A thorough discussion of the alternative and natural neuropathy treatments is beyond this book's scope. It would require a dedicated chapter on neuropathy treatment. However, a good place to start is with 500 mg of Acetyl L-carnitine 3 times a day combined with 500 mg of Alpha Lipoic Acid twice a day. I have had moderate neuropathy in my feet and hands for over 10 years and have found that this combination has reduced my symptoms by 50% and stopped the progression of the symptoms during the past 10 years. If this works for you, you should begin to see results with this combination in about 60 days.

Homocysteine & ED

High homocysteine levels are commonly associated with heart disease, stroke, and dementia. Common symptoms include fatigue, pins and needles in the hands and feet, dizziness, and mood changes. While free testosterone, DHEA, and SHBG are often discussed as potential causes of ED, the link between high homocysteine levels and ED is less well-known. It is less common for men with ED to be tested for high homocysteine levels. However, a growing body of scientific research has established a link between high homocysteine levels and ED. A 2018 meta-analysis by Sansome and colleagues of nine studies involving 1,320 men showed a direct link between high homocysteine levels and ED. (12) A diet high in meat, protein, and dairy can raise homocysteine levels. However, a deficiency in or low levels of the B vitamins B12, B6, and folate (folic acid) is the most common cause of high homocysteine levels. The absorption of B12 from diet, in particular, declines with age. The supplement maker Superior Source® markets a sublingual combination of these three B vitamins with 1000 mcg of B12, 2 mg of B6, and 800 mcg of folic acid. Sublingual vitamins enhance absorption. The B6 in this product is only 117.7% of RDA, which is important for men with chronic prostatitis because very high levels of B6 can cause dysuria.

Major Risk Factors: Obesity, Smoking, and Alcohol

These risk factors have been extensively studied and proven to contribute to ED. Developing and implementing treatment programs for severe obesity, heavy smoking, and heavy drinking, particularly alcoholism, exceeds the scope of this book. You should collaborate with your doctors to manage these risk factors. Obesity in general and abdominal obesity in particular are associated with a significantly higher risk of ED. Studies indicate that reducing obesity is linked with lower rates of ED. Smoking is also associated with much higher rates of ED, and men who quit smoking have lower rates of ED. Heavy regular use of alcohol, defined here as having more than 2 drinks per day or 14 drinks per week, is linked to ED. Whereas moderate use of alcohol, less than 2 drinks per day, may lead to a slight improvement in cardiovascular health and

CHAPTER 9
Erectile Dysfunction and Chronic Prostatitis

possibly erectile function. This was the consensus based on several studies as recently as 8 years ago. (5) However, more recent research argues that there is no safe level of alcohol use for our health, including cardiovascular health, and that any level of alcohol consumption is harmful to cardiovascular health and, by implication, erectile function, especially in the long run. (6) The remaining argument for moderate drinking, 1 or 2 drinks occasionally, maybe that it relaxes men and therefore helps with overall success leading up to sex. There is some limited research to back this up, but it's difficult to measure and study. This may be a case of using your individual judgment and determining what works for you. If you have implemented the Prostatitis 360 Protocol at this point, you will have stopped drinking on a regular daily or weekly basis, stopped smoking, and reduced your level of obesity. If not, addressing these risk factors will, in most cases, help with your ED.

Depression & Chronic Stress

There is a strong link between chronic stress, depression, and erectile dysfunction. In approximately 20% of men, emotional and psychological factors are the main cause of ED. In the remaining 80%, physical factors are the main cause of ED. Men with chronic stress, anxiety, and depression have a higher risk of developing ED. A 2018 meta-analysis of 48 studies by Lin and colleagues that examined the link between depression and ED found that depression results in a 39% increase in the likelihood of developing ED. (7) The reasons why depression increases the likelihood of developing ED are not fully understood, but it's believed that depression has emotional consequences, such as lower sexual self-confidence, and physical consequences, such as lower testosterone, that impact ED. Perhaps the best evidence of this link between depression and ED is a 2014 review and meta-analysis by Schmidt and colleagues that found that a combination treatment of ED drugs and treatment for depression was more effective than ED drugs alone in treating ED. If you're struggling with depression and ED, it's important to treat both conditions, and in the process of treating each one, you're likely to see an improvement in both conditions.

Chronic stress is also strongly linked with ED. A 2023 study of men between 18 and 60 by Xiao and colleagues found that 65% of men with chronic stress/anxiety had ED. It's also interesting to note that the study found poor sleep and lack of exercise to be common among men struggling with depression, anxiety, and ED. As in the case of ED and depression treatment, stress management treatment can play an important role in improving ED symptoms. An 8/20/14 study by Kalatzidou and colleagues found that an 8-week stress management program combined with the ED drug Tadalafil (Cialis) was more effective than Tadalafil alone. (9)

One of the many challenges for men with chronic prostatitis, ED, depression, or chronic stress is that they create a three-part vicious cycle. Chronic prostatitis can lead to depression, chronic stress, and ED. Chronic stress and depression often lead to or make ED worse, and ED, in turn, makes depression and chronic stress worse in a vicious cycle. The way to break the cycle is to treat all three conditions and use combination treatments. In the context of the typical HMO or PPO healthcare that most Americans have, it may be that the only way you can develop and implement combination treatments is to do it yourself by seeking treatment for ED and depression, for example, independently but at the same time. As discussed in Chapter 3, we do not have an integrative or holistic approach to health care in the US. It is highly unlikely that your

CHAPTER 9
Erectile Dysfunction and Chronic Prostatitis

urologist or primary care doctor will develop and implement an 8-week or 12-week combination treatment plan, for example, that combines stress management with Tadalafil to treat your ED.

The Role of Lifestyle and Diet

A wide range of lifestyle and diet factors have been extensively studied and proven to play a direct role in leading to low-grade inflammation, low free testosterone, and decreased nitrate nitric oxide (NO) availability and activity, all of which combine to lead to ED. Free testosterone and nitric oxide play a critical role in the ability to establish and maintain an erection strong enough for successful sexual intercourse.

Exercise: Important Role in Treating ED

A sedentary lifestyle is widely regarded as a major risk factor for erectile dysfunction and has been validated by extensive scientific research. Starting and maintaining a lifetime commitment to a regular aerobic exercise program is the single most important thing you can do that doesn't require drugs to treat and manage your ED. This is regardless of whether you have mild, moderate, or severe ED. A regular aerobic exercise program has a wide range of emotional, psychological, and physical health benefits in addition to improving your ED, including lowering stress, obesity, hypertension, cholesterol, and many more. These benefits don't exist in a vacuum but work together synergistically in a virtuous cycle that, among other things, improves your ED symptoms over time. In fact, if you have led a sedentary lifestyle, a regular aerobic exercise program may be the single most important thing you can do to improve your overall health and the quality of your life.

An ideal aerobic exercise program has been well-defined and extensively researched. It's important to start slowly and implement the program in consultation with your doctor, ideally under the supervision of a trained expert, during the first six months. Two of the best forms of aerobic exercise are power walking on a treadmill and swimming laps in a pool. Using a treadmill that has a heart rate monitor is a great way to start by building up from walking to power-walking. Another excellent option, especially for men over 50, is swimming laps because it puts a great deal less stress on the joints. It also has the advantage of being an excellent form of exercise for the entire body. Regardless of how active you may have been in your teens or 20s, if you are over 40 and have been physically inactive for a decade or more, you may be surprised to find how slow you must start. You may find that even if you swim slowly, you can't complete a second lap in a 25-meter pool or walk, much less jog, for more than 5 or 10 minutes. This is normal. It's important not to be discouraged by the initial slow start and progress.

The Aerobic Exercise Program

Once you choose the best form of exercise for you. The exercise program you follow is straightforward and has been proven by extensive research. The basic program is:

- 160 minutes of aerobic exercise per week
- 40 minutes a day, 4 days a week
- Raised heart rate & breeding for 40 minutes

It may take any 3 to 6 months to reach this goal. Take your time and reach this target at a comfortable pace that works for you. This exercise program is proven and well-researched. A 2018 meta-analysis of 10 studies by Larsen and colleagues is a good example. The study reported that across all 10 studies in the meta-analysis, the improvement ranged from 18% to 86%, with an average

CHAPTER 9
Erectile Dysfunction and Chronic Prostatitis

improvement of over 40%. The authors concluded: "Overall, weekly exercise of 160 minutes for 6 months contributes to decreasing erectile problems in men with ED caused by physical inactivity, obesity, hypertension, metabolic syndrome, and/or cardiovascular diseases." (10) Metabolic syndrome is a condition that includes a combination of risk factors specific to cardiovascular disease. These include abdominal obesity, high blood pressure, impaired fasting glucose, high triglyceride levels, and low HDL cholesterol levels. It's important to be patient. In most studies, it takes 6 months to see the full benefit of an aerobic exercise program.

Diet

If you have more severe ED, diet alone, as in the case of aerobic exercise, is normally not enough to return to normal erectile function. The goal is to use lifestyle changes, aerobic exercise, diet, and supplements to minimize the dosage of ED drugs that you'll need to achieve a normal, healthy sex life. Ideally, you will rely solely on daily 5 mg Tadalafil to minimize or largely avoid the side effects of stronger doses of Tadalafil, Viagra, and similar ED drugs. If, on the other hand, you have mild to moderate ED lifestyle changes, diet, and supplements alone, or perhaps in the case of moderate ED, 2.5 mg daily Tadalafil may be enough.

The best diet for optimal sexual health for men at any age, including men over 60, is the Mediterranean diet. This diet has been extensively researched and has consistently proven to be the most effective in helping men prevent and improve ED. The Mediterranean diet is defined in almost all studies as a diet high in vegetables, fruits, nuts, legumes, and fish, as well as avoiding or limiting red and processed meats. Common legumes include beans, peas, lentils, chickpeas, and peanuts. Processed meats include sausages, cold cuts, and other highly processed meat made with additives, preservatives, and salt. One of the most authoritative long-term studies of the Mediterranean diet was published in 2020 by Bauer and colleagues. The Bauer study followed 21,469 men between the ages of 40 and 75 from 1986 to 2014. The study divided the men into quintiles (5 groups of 20%) based on their adherence to the Mediterranean diet. The top 20% group with the highest adherence to the Mediterranean diet were the least likely to have ED. This applied to both men under 60 and over 60. (13) A study done in 2021 by Angelis and colleagues found that the Mediterranean diet improved erectile function in several important ways, including better blood flow and exercise capacity, higher testosterone, healthier arteries, and lower hypertension. In middle-aged men, blood flow, testosterone, and exercise capacity decline. (14) A meta-analysis done in 2017 by Di Francesco and colleagues found that the Mediterranean diet lowers high cholesterol. Blood pressure and glucose levels while increasing antioxidant defenses and raising arginine levels, which raises NO levels. Raising and maintaining high NO levels is one of the most important aspects of healthy erectile function. (15)

There are some important guidelines to follow in implementing the Mediterranean Diet. It's important to have several servings of fresh fruits and vegetables every day. If you have three meals a day, you should have a fruit and vegetable with each meal at a minimum as a starting point. Unless out of season, all the fruits and vegetables should be fresh. The general guidelines for a healthy diet in the US call for two servings of fish per week. The ideal Mediterranean Diet for ED involves four servings of fish in addition to sardines and anchovies, for example, used as appetizers and side dishes on a daily basis. In the classic Mediterranean diet, fruit is used as the main dessert, and desserts made with added sugar (cakes, cookies, etc.) are used sparingly for special occasions and holidays. Added sugar

CHAPTER 9
Erectile Dysfunction and Chronic Prostatitis

and sugary drinks are among the worst foods for ED and should be removed from the diet entirely, especially if you have severe ED. One of the keys to the Mediterranean Diet is the use of extra virgin olive oil (EVOO) as the primary cooking fat, replacing butter, vegetable oil, and other fats. EVOO is also used as the main salad dressing alone or combined with a small amount of red wine vinegar. Mediterranean cuisines use herbs such as oregano and basil for seasoning, largely replacing salt. Many men with ED have hypertension or borderline hypertension. Removing salt from the diet of men with hypertension is one of the most important dietary recommendations for managing hypertension. Salt is widely used in packaged foods. Removing salt from your diet involves a commitment to cooking with whole fresh foods.

The Mediterranean Diet is a dramatic change from the "American Diet." If you're a middle-aged American man with ED who grew up on and has eaten an American diet all your adult life, adopting a Mediterranean diet will involve a dramatic change in your diet, including how you shop for and prepare food. The transition to a Mediterranean diet will be difficult for most men and require adapting to a whole range of new foods eaten daily. This transition may require six months or more. It's important to remain patient. The many health benefits go beyond helping to reverse ED to a transformation of overall health and quality of life in your middle age and the rest of your life.

The Prostatitis 360 Protocol Diet is the Mediterranean Diet with some additional changes and fine-tuning to remove tomato-based foods, citrus, spicy foods, acidic foods, and alcohol. Moderate drinking of red wine with meals, for example, is traditionally part of the Mediterranean Diet. The Prostatitis 360 Protocol Diet is not a new, separate, or alternative diet but a modified version of the scientifically proven Mediterranean Diet.

ED Superfoods

In addition to following the guidelines for a Mediterranean diet, there are specific fruits, vegetables, and nuts that are superfoods in terms of their ability to reverse and enhance erectile function. These superfoods fall into several categories, including foods that impact NO, testosterone, L-Arginine, and antioxidant levels. Nitrate, L-citrulline, and L-arginine-rich foods enhance Nitrate Oxide (NO) production in the body. One of the keys to a healthy erection. L-citrulline enhances the conversion of L-arginine into NO. Zinc increases Testosterone levels. Studies show that regularly eating certain foods rich in flavonoids, such as berries, is associated with a lower incidence of ED. Finally, enhanced blood flow is important for lowering ED.

Nitrate-Rich Foods
Pomegranates & pomegranate juice
Beets & beet juice
Dark leafy greens: spinach, romaine, arugula, etc.

L-Arginine Rich Foods
Oatmeal
Legumes (beans, lentils, etc.)
Nuts & Seeds

Foods that Enhance Blood Flow
Pistachios
Walnuts
Hazelnuts
Almonds

Flavonoid-Rich Foods
Berries: blueberries, blackberries, raspberries

CHAPTER 9
Erectile Dysfunction and Chronic Prostatitis

Onions
Garlic
Tea (caffeine-free)
Apples

Note: Dark chocolate (70% or more) is normally part of a list like this but is excluded here because it's high in caffeine and, therefore, excluded from the diet of men with chronic prostatitis.

Foods Rich in Citrulline
Watermelon
Cantaloupe
Cucumber

Foods Rich in Zinc
Oysters
Shellfish
Eggs
Chickpeas
Pumpkin Seeds

The foods in each of the categories above are commonly available and easily included in the daily diet of men with ED. Incorporating some of the foods in each category can boost the benefits of the Mediterranean diet in reversing ED.

Supplements for ED
For men with severe ED, supplements alone or in combination with diet, exercise, and lifestyle changes will not restore normal healthy erectile function. The goal here, as in the case of diet and exercise, is to minimize the use of ED medications to the lowest necessary

dose and, therefore, avoid or lower the side effects of these ED drugs. The goal, once you fully implement the diet and lifestyle changes and allow time for supplements to work, is to rely on 5mg daily Tadalafil as the primary ED prescription medication. If, on the other hand, you have mild ED, and even in some cases moderate ED, it may be that supplements, diet, and exercise alone may be enough to fully restore normal healthy erectile function, especially if you're under 60.

There are over two dozen different supplements that are used to "treat" or are believed to play a role in reversing ED. There are, in fact, only three supplements that have been proven in multiple rigorous scientific RCT studies to be effective in treating ED. The three supplements are Arginine, Panax Ginseng, and Tribulus Terrestris. There are also some add-on supplements that are combined with these three to enhance their effectiveness. None of these alone or in combination treat severe ED. All of these supplements treat "Mild and Mild-Moderate" ED based on the IIEF scale, and most medical research done on ED using supplements involves testing of men in these two categories. The International Index of Erectile Function Questionnaire, or IIEF, is the most widely used measure of the level of erectile function used in medical research. The IIEF consists of 15 questions rated on a 0 to 5 or one to five scale with a total score ranging from 22-25 is No ED, 17-21 is Mild ED, 12-16 is Mild-Moderate ED, 8-11 is Moderate ED, and 5-7 is Severe ED. The IIEF Questionnaire is available for download by searching for "IIEF pdf." If you have not completed the questionnaire, you should complete it now and use it to measure your progress as you implement various ED treatments. If you have mild or mild-moderate ED, you may be able to treat your ED with a combination of supplements and diet and lifestyle changes without the need to use prescription ED medications or very low-dose

CHAPTER 9
Erectile Dysfunction and Chronic Prostatitis

versions of these medications. This is important because prescription ED medications, especially at higher doses, can involve potentially severe side effects. Approximately 30% of men with ED are unable to use prescription ED drugs because of side effects. If you have severe ED, you may be able to treat your condition with diet and lifestyle changes and a combination of supplements and lower-dose versions of ED drugs.

L-Arginine

L-arginine is the most widely studied supplement for ED, alone or in combination with other supplements or ED drugs. It's also the most widely used ED supplement, usually in combination with other supplements. It's important to note that a study done by Petre and colleagues in 2023 found that most commercial products sold as combinations of ED supplements do not have a high enough dose of the most effective ED supplements, including L-arginine, Panax Ginseng, Tribulus Terrestris, and Pycnogenol, to be effective. (15) This is especially true in the case of L-Arginine, which requires between 3000 and 6000 mg daily and is the high end of that range for most men. Many commercial ED supplement combinations consist of 6 to 12 or more supplements, many of which have weak or no evidence of effective ED treatments. The most effective way to use supplements for ED is to build your own combination using the individual supplements and adjust the dose of each supplement as needed, all based on proven scientific evidence of effectiveness for treating ED. You can use this guide to determine which supplements and doses may be right for you. There is an element of trial and error in selecting the optimal supplement and dose for you. The same is true with ED drugs; your doctor experiments with different ED drugs and doses to determine what works best for you.

A 2019 meta-analysis by Rhim and colleagues of L-arginine alone or in combination with other supplements involving 10 studies concluded that it provides significant improvement with only minor side effects. (16) A study by Manfra and colleagues in 2022 using 6000 milligrams daily of L-Arginine for three months involving primarily men with mild-moderate ED found that 74% of the men improved and 20% of the men reported having no ED at the end of the Study. This study is important because it overcomes many of the drawbacks and limitations of earlier studies, which do not use a high enough dose, are too short (typically two months or less), do not include older men, and do not include men with severe ED. This study included men aged 20 to 75 with severe ED. It found that arginine alone, using a very high dose for three months, was not effective for men with severe ED. (17) L-citrulline is an amino acid similar to L-arginine that enhances NO in the body in part by improving the conversion of L-arginine into NO. There is some limited research that demonstrates L-citrulline is similar to L-arginine in improving ED symptoms, and one study done in Japan shows similar results for the combination of L-arginine and L-citrulline. A study done by Barassi and colleagues in 2016 makes a more compelling case for adding L-citrulline to L-arginine to enhance its effectiveness in treating ED. The study compared men with severe and mild ED and measured their levels of L-arginine and L-citrulline. It found that men with severe ED had 17% less L-arginine and 13% less L-citrulline (18). Studies also show that taking them together is more effective in improving NO levels than either alone. Most studies use 1000 to 3000 mg daily of L-citrulline and 3000 to 6000 mg daily of L-arginine. Depending on your level of ED, using these doses of the two supplements may be the best way to increase the benefit of L-arginine for ED treatment and, if

CHAPTER 9
Erectile Dysfunction and Chronic Prostatitis

you have severe ED, to help with lowering a possible deficiency in L-arginine and L-citrulline.

L-arginine & Pycnogenol®

L-arginine and Pycnogenol® is the most widely researched supplement combination for ED, including 5 RCT studies and three studies of a commercial product called Prelox® that uses this combination and one study of L-arginine combined with L-Citrulline and Pycnogenol®. A meta-analysis done by Tian and colleagues of three studies for men with mild-moderate ED reported: "There were significant differences in International Index of Erectile Function (IIEF) scores (erectile domain), Intercourse satisfaction scores, orgasmic function scores, overall satisfaction scores, and sexual desire scores, between the combination treatment group and the control group." (19) Perhaps the most widely quoted study of this combination was done by Stanislavov in 2003. In this three-month study using 1700 mg of L-arginine and 120 mg of Pycnogenol®, the author reported that after three months, 92.5% of the men had normal erections. This would be an impressive outcome if not for the fact that the men studied were between 25 and 45. Most men with ED, especially men with ED that is more than mild, are over 45. Similar results have not been replicated in middle-aged and older men. A study was done in 2015, also by Stanislavov and a colleague, combined L-arginine and Pycnogenol® with L-citrulline and Robuvit®. Robuvit® is a commercially available polyphenol called Roburins, which is a French oak wood extract. While there are no scientific studies to validate it, it is believed to have, among many other benefits, the improvement of ED in older men. In this study, this combination restored erectile function to normal for men with moderate ED after one month based on the IIEF scale. (21) Unfortunately, there have been no other follow-up studies since

2015 to validate these impressive results. Based on the studies that have been done, the dose for treating ED, especially more severe ED, is 3000 to 6000 mg L-arginine, 1500 to 3000 mg of L-citrulline, 120 milligrams of Pycnogenol®, and 200 mg of Robuvit® as the daily dose. In terms of treatment cost, L-arginine and L-citrulline are inexpensive. Robuvit® is a little more expensive, but the daily dose is only one capsule. Pycnogenol is expensive, but there may be a very good, inexpensive alternative in the form of grape seed extract or GSE. GSE is believed to have the same active ingredients and may actually have some advantages compared to Pycnogenol. GSE has been studied in combination with other supplements for treating ED, but unfortunately, there are no studies that do a head-to-head comparison between GSE and Pycnogenol® for treating ED. Finally, there have been some other studies of L-arginine combined with other supplements. Notably, a 2008 RCT study the combined L-arginine with SOD and GSE, and a 2012 RCT study the combined L-arginine with niacin and PLC. Both studies showed some significant improvement, especially the 2008 study, but there have been no follow-up studies of these combinations to validate the results. The takeaway on the use of L-arginine and Pycnogenol® when combined with L-citrulline and the diet and lifestyle changes

discussed above is that, in many cases, it should be an effective treatment for mild ED and may in some cases be effective in mild-moderate ED on the IIEF scale. There are no studies, however, on the effectiveness of a complete optimal diet lifestyle and supplement protocol for moderate and severe ED. The complete optimal program would include the diet and lifestyle changes discussed above with 6000 mg of arginine, 3000 mg of citrulline, and 120 mg of Pycnogenol® or 250 mg of grape seed extract.

L-arginine and 5 mg Tadalafil

Arginine and 5 mg Tadalafil are the most widely studied and used combination of a supplement with a prescription ED medication. Tadalafil 5 milligram is the most widely used daily dose ED medication. It is primarily designed to treat mild and moderate ED. It has proven to have few and minor side effects compared to higher-dose, on-demand ED medications. Numerous studies done during the past 20 years have consistently shown that adding L-arginine to Tadalafil, as well as other ED medications, is more effective than ED medication treatment alone. A 2023 meta-analysis of four studies done by Wibisono and colleagues reported that adding between 2500 mg and 5000 mg of arginine to 5 mg daily of Tadalafil was more effective than Tadalafil alone in treating mild and moderate ED. (22) This meta-analysis and a study done by Gallo and colleagues in 2020 concluded that the combination of 2500 mg arginine and 5 mg Tadalafil was not effective in treating severe ED. (23) However, studies of the combination of 5000 mg L-arginine and 5mg Tadalafil have proven to be more effective in treating severe ED. The most compelling of these studies involved a study done by Hamd and colleagues in 2020, which used this combination for men with ED over 60 with an average age of 66. The study found that after just six weeks, there was a "dramatic improvement" in ED using the Sexual Health Inventory for Men or SHIM score and a significant increase in testosterone levels. This study is important because the prevalence and severity of ED increase dramatically after age 60 and is more difficult to treat successfully. (24) While many of the men in this study saw a dramatic improvement in their ED, not all of them experienced a return to normal erectile function. We can only speculate about the impact of implementing a completely optimized diet, lifestyle, and supplement program combined with 5 mg Tadalafil, including 6000 mg arginine, 3000 mg citrulline, and 120 mg Pycnogenol® or 250 mg of GSE, but it's reasonable to assume that this complete program would significantly improve the results. Finally, it's important to note that this was an unusually short study, lasting just six weeks, while most studies last 12 weeks or longer. Once again, it's reasonable to assume, based on the outcomes from longer studies, that the improvement reported in this study would continue to increase after 9 and 12 weeks.

Severe ED & Higher Dose Tadalafil

For men with severe ED who don't respond to the program discussed above, the next step up is to use a 10 mg or 20 mg dose of Tadalafil taken three times a week or every other day. Studies of 10 and 20 mg Tadalafil alone show that 10 mg Tadalafil is nearly as effective as 20 mg Tadalafil and is effective in treating severe ED. Once again, it's reasonable to assume that adding diet, lifestyle, and the three-supplement program discussed above to 10 mg Tadalafil would significantly improve the results and perhaps not require using 20 mg tadalafil. The goal is to use the lowest effective dose of Tadalafil to minimize any potentially serious side effects. Studies of 10 and 20 mg Tadalafil show that they are effective in treating moderate and severe ED with a high overall satisfaction rate. The ability to engage in spontaneous sex restores normal sexual self-confidence as well as overall self-confidence over time. This, in turn, increases, for reasons that are not fully understood, total and presumably free testosterone and creates a virtuous cycle of improving erectile function and overall sexual health. Finally, for men with severe ED who don't see immediate results, it's important to recognize that it takes six months or longer to see the full benefits of the diet and aerobic exercise programs discussed above. It's also important to work with your doctors to treat any underlying conditions that may be contributing to your severe ED. These not

CHAPTER 9
Erectile Dysfunction and Chronic Prostatitis

only include serious conditions such as heart disease, diabetes, and metabolic syndrome but also early-stage conditions such as prediabetes and prehypertension.

Additional Supplements for ED

There are several additional supplements that have been RCT-studied for ED alone and in combination with other supplements and ED drugs for mild and moderate ED. The number of rigorous scientific studies for these additional supplements is much more limited compared to arginine alone or in combination with other supplements and ED drugs. However, for men with mild and moderate ED, there may be viable alternatives if arginine is not effective, either alone or in combination with other supplements and ED drugs. There are 4 additional supplements that stand out in terms of the number of studies and effectiveness. They are Tribulus Terrestris, Ginseng, and Yohimbe, as well as Propionyl L-carnitine or PLC as a combination supplement used with ED drugs.

Tribulus Terrestris

A review of 4 RCT studies of Tribulus Terrestris shows that it is effective for mild and mild-moderate ED on the IIEF scale. One study in particular reported that for men with mild ED, a dose of 500 mg 3x daily restored mild ED to normal erectile function after just four weeks. The number of studies is limited, but they all show similar positive results from mild and mild-moderate ED. The dosages studied ranged from 800 mg 2x 400 mg daily to 1500 mg 3x 500 mg daily. There are no studies of Tribulus Terrestris combined with other supplements or ED drugs.

Panax Ginseng

Several studies of Panax Ginseng, aka Korean Ginseng, reported significant improvement for men with mild to mild-moderate ED. One study (de Andrade, 2007) with particularly impressive results using 3000 mg (1000 mg 3x daily) of Panax Ginseng for men with mild to mild-moderate ED reported that 66.6% of the men saw significant improvement with an average point increase on the IIEF scale of 4.6 from 16.4 to 21.0 or a 21.9% improvement. To put these results in perspective, 16.4 is the top of the mild-moderate range, and 21.0 is the top of the mild range, just one point below normal erectile function, which is 22 to 25 on the IIEF scale. Several other studies using a total daily dosage of 1400 to 3000 mg divided into 3 to 4 doses during the day have reported fairly similar results. There is one study in Japan (Yamaguchi, 2018) of men with severe ED who reported significant improvement after 12 weeks of Panax Ginseng. Unfortunately, this is the only study of men with severe ED. On the other hand, some other studies of the effectiveness of Panax Ginseng as a treatment for ED are mixed. Notably, a meta-analysis (Lee, 2021) of 9 studies concluded that Panax Ginseng had "a trivial effect on erectile dysfunction". (26) There is no clear explanation for these discrepancies between studies. Men considering Panax Ginseng as an alternative to L-arginine should be aware that it may not be effective. Unlike arginine, Panax ginseng has not been extensively studied in combination with other supplements, and there are no studies combining it with ED drugs. There's only one study of Ginseng combined with vitamin E and one study that uses the combination of Ginseng with Rutin and Moringa, with both studies reporting significant but not dramatic improvement.

CHAPTER 9
Erectile Dysfunction and Chronic Prostatitis

Yohimbe / Yohimbine Warning

Yohimbine has been extensively studied for the treatment of ED alone but primarily in combination with other supplements, most notably arginine. It has been widely studied, with extensive research done in the 1980s and 1990s, including a meta-analysis completed in 1998. Studies during the past 40 years have consistently shown that Yohimbine provides a significant benefit as the treatment for mild and moderate ED. Several of these studies involved very high doses of 6000 mg taken as a single dose rather than divided into 2 or 3 doses. As a result of these studies, 6000 mg of Yohimbine has been widely recommended, often in conjunction with 6000 mg of arginine, as a treatment for ED. In the US, supplements like Yohimbine are not regulated, and studies have shown that in some cases, Yohimbine supplements have higher and, in some cases, much higher doses of Yohimbine than disclosed on the product labels. This sets the stage for growing concerns about the dangers of Yohimbine. In recent years, there has been growing evidence of the potential for serious side effects from the use of Yohimbine, especially at high doses. Yet, it's high doses of yohimbine that are often recommended to treat even mild and moderate ED. Reports of the serious health dangers of Yohimbine include heart attacks, seizures, kidney failure, anxiety attacks, and liver damage. Some of the alarming side effects include rapid heart rate, elevated high blood pressure, and anxiety. Individuals with heart disease, high blood pressure, kidney disease, and mental disorders are advised not to use Yohimbine. In the US, the FDA has had reports of seizures and kidney failure, while in Europe, the EU has warned against using Yohimbine, and Germany has banned it. The entire rationale of using supplements for treating ED is that supplements are intended to be safe alternatives to ED drugs for mild and mild-moderate ED and enhancements to the effectiveness of low-dose 5 mg and 10 mg Tadalafil to avoid higher doses and more dangerous ED drugs in the case of moderate and severe ED. Regardless of how rare serious side effects may be, there is no rationale for using Yohimbine, especially since there are proven, extensively tested, and safe alternatives such as arginine and arginine combinations that are more effective.

Other Supplements & Treatments

There are several supplements that help specific ED-related issues, as well as new and emerging supplements that may be additional treatment options in the future.

- **Propynyl L-carnitine / PLC**: PLC has demonstrated promising results in combination with several ED drugs, including Sildenafil (Viagra) alone or combined with Acetyl L-Carnitine, Tadalafil, and Vardenafil combined with L-arginine and nicotinic acid. PLC has also been studied with arginine and niacin, with a small but significant improvement.

- **Resveratrol:** Resveratrol is a new emerging potential treatment for ED that targets oxidative stress and acts as a SIRT1 inhibitor. It is at the animal study stage where it has shown promise in diabetic and age-related ED, as well as a potential combination with Tadalafil.

- **Chrysin:** Chrysin is a powerful natural flavonoid inhibitor of aromatase. Aromatase converts testosterone into estrogen in the body, thereby lowering the level of testosterone. Excess estrogen is a common problem among aging men. Chrysin increases free testosterone by inhibiting aromatase.

CHAPTER 9
Erectile Dysfunction and Chronic Prostatitis

Men over 45 with ED should have their estradiol level tested. Dose: 500 mg/d.

- **Nettle Root Extract:** A hormone called sex hormone binding globulin, or SHBG, controls the level of free testosterone. The testosterone-binding free testosterone-lowering action of SHBG increases dramatically after age 45 – by 40% on average – and is associated with age-related ED. Nettle Root Extract interferes with the free testosterone-lowering action of SHBG and, therefore, increases free testosterone. The supplements zinc, magnesium, and boron, as well as aerobic exercise and a low sugar/high fiber diet, also help, but Nettle Root Extract is the most powerful. Men over 45 should have their SHBG level tested. Dose: 500 mg one to three times a day.

- **Fenugreek & Ashwagandha:** Several studies, including a meta-analysis (Smith, 2019), have shown that these two supplements stand out in terms of their ability to increase total and, perhaps most importantly, free testosterone in men between 40 and 70. Fenugreek has been shown to increase testosterone by 22% to 46% and Ashwagandha by 14% to 20%. Other helpful supplements include zinc, vitamin D3, and magnesium glycinate. Dose: 500 mg/d for Fenugreek and 600 mg/d for Ashwagandha.

- **DHEA:** Low levels of DHEA can result in low testosterone. DHEA begins to decline gradually after age 30, and DHEA deficiency is common among men over 50. If there is a deficiency, supplementing with DHEA can increase testosterone levels. Men with chronic prostatitis, however, must exercise caution because supplementing with more than 30 mg can cause Dysuria. Men over 45 with ED should test for DHEA levels and re-test after supplementing. Dose: 10 to 20 mg daily taken in the morning.

We have discussed a wide range of steps you can take to diagnose and treat your erectile dysfunction. However, there are three basic numbers you should know at the start of the process and test every 6 to 12 months. You should know your total testosterone, free testosterone, and SHGB levels. Once you have these three numbers and you monitor them on a regular basis, you and your doctor have a good basic starting point for managing your ED.

CHAPTER 10
Chronic Prostatitis and Depression

It's important to recognize at the outset that this chapter is a departure from the rest of the book. The treatment of depression, especially serious depression, is very different from the treatment of the other major symptoms of chronic prostatitis. The primary treatments of chronic prostatitis are based on alternative rather than conventional medicine. Conventional medical treatment has a role to play, but it's a secondary role. The primary treatment for chronic prostatitis involves the use of a range of natural and alternative treatments. Indeed, the Chronic Prostatitis 360 Protocol was developed, and this book was written in response to the fact that conventional medicine, as practiced in the US, is largely ineffective in treating chronic prostatitis.

When it comes to depression, however, it's very different. The treatment of depression relies primarily on the use of conventional medicine. There is a role for complementary treatments and what conventional medicine calls Complimentary Alternative Medicine or CAM, but it's a secondary role. The treatment of depression is very complex and difficult, but conventional medicine is successful in many cases. A wide range of complementary treatment approaches can help, but there is no proven viable alternative to conventional medicine for treating depression. Therefore, if you have depression, the first step is always to work with a mental health professional, typically a psychiatrist, to treat your depression.

The treatment of depression involves several unique challenges. There is still a stigma in our society around the treatment of mental health issues, including depression. Many of us are reluctant to discuss depression symptoms, especially serious depression. Men are socialized from an early age to be "tough," which can result in some men seeing professional mental health care as a sign of weakness when, in fact, it is a sign of wisdom, strength, and character. Depression is a serious medical condition and must be taken seriously by immediately seeking professional mental health care. It's very important not to engage in self-diagnosis. A doctor who specializes in treating depression should be the one to help you determine how serious your depression is- mild, moderate, or serious depression and work with you to determine the right treatment program for your situation. If you have serious depression, it may be very difficult to treat your chronic prostatitis symptoms unless you treat you are depression, especially serious depression.

Chronic prostatitis is a chronic pain disorder. Chronic pain is, in fact, the defining symptom of the condition. Depression is one of the most common side effects of chronic pain disorders. Chronic prostatitis has a profound impact not only on physical health but also on emotional and psychological health. Men with chronic prostatitis struggle with various levels of chronic stress, anxiety, and depression. High levels of chronic stress, anxiety, and depression are common, including serious or clinical depression. Stress and anxiety impact chronic prostatitis symptoms and treatment, but

CHAPTER 10
Chronic Prostatitis and Depression

serious depression makes it particularly difficult to successfully treat the condition. Therefore, the treatment of stress, anxiety, depression, and serious depression, in particular, plays an important role in the successful treatment of chronic prostatitis.

Depression

Studies done during the past 25 years (Collins 2001, Chung 2011, Krieger 2016) consistently show that approximately 50% of men with chronic prostatitis are diagnosed with severe depression. A recent comprehensive and detailed meta-analysis of 10 studies done in 2020 by Huang and colleagues reported that 46% of men with chronic prostatitis have serious depression, and 26% were diagnosed with pain catastrophizing. **(1)** This study is particularly important because it identified the sub-segment of men diagnosed with pain catastrophizing.

The treatment of depression and the pain of chronic prostatitis is made particularly difficult by pain catastrophizing, which characterizes how individuals respond to chronic pain. Catastrophizing is a set of three attitudes towards or feelings about pain: 1. Rumination or worrying ("can't keep it out of my mind"), 2. Magnifying ("makes me think about other pains"), and 3. Helpless ("there is nothing I can do") when experiencing or anticipating pain" **(2).** Catastrophizing makes pain worse by increasing the perception of pain. It also makes urinary symptoms, depression, quality of life, and overall disability worse. It is believed to develop in stages, starting with rumination and magnifying and leading to helplessness, which may make the helpless catastrophizing stage the most difficult to treat.

The pain of chronic prostatitis, depression, and pain catastrophizing creates a vicious cycle that can be difficult to break. Pain severity is the single greatest predictor of serious depression in men with chronic prostatitis. In most cases, the path to depression starts with severe chronic prostatitis pain, and the best way to break this vicious cycle is to start the process of treating the pain until it's dramatically reduced. Treating depression does help, but unless the pain severity is dramatically reduced, it's unlikely to break the cycle by itself.

A detailed or nuanced discussion of the treatment of depression is beyond the scope of this book. If you have depression or suspect you have depression, whether it's mild, moderate, or serious, your focus should be on working with a mental health professional to treat your depression. It's not necessary to extensively study the treatment of depression in general. However, it is wise to understand and have some background about the treatment of depression in men with chronic prostatitis. Your doctor may have a great deal of expertise in the treatment of depression but may be less knowledgeable about treating depression in men with chronic prostatitis. What follows is a discussion of the treatment of depression that is focused on what we know about treating depression in men with chronic prostatitis. There is, unfortunately, not a great deal of rigorous scientific research on the treatment of serious depression in men with chronic prostatitis. The available information can be very helpful. The two most common treatments for serious depression, CBT and antidepressants, have also been studied as treatments for chronic prostatitis-related depression.

CHAPTER 10
Chronic Prostatitis and Depression

Cognitive Behavior Therapy (CBT) and Depression

Since the early 2000s, two of the most prominent experts in the field of chronic prostatitis treatment research in North America, Dr J Curtis Nickel and Dr Daniel Shoskes, have recommended psychotherapy to treat depression and pain catastrophizing in men with chronic prostatitis. (3) However, since then, there has been limited scientific research on the effectiveness of psychotherapy for the treatment of depression and pain catastrophizing in men with chronic prostatitis. A 2008 study by Nickel and colleagues presented an 8-week cognitive behavior therapy (CBT) treatment program for depression and pain catastrophizing designed for men with chronic prostatitis. The researchers reported that after eight weeks, the program provided significant benefits and reduced depression and pain catastrophizing. (3) A study done by Kwon and colleagues in 2013 reported significant improvement in depression and pain catastrophizing after implementing a psychotherapy program. (4) A 2022 meta-analysis by Sone-Wi Li and colleagues reviewed four studies in which cognitive behavior therapy (CBT) was used to treat men with chronic prostatitis and showed significant benefits. (5) A small study by Trip and colleagues done in 2011 reported positive outcomes, but it only involved 11 men with moderate chronic prostatitis symptoms. (6) A 2024 review by Lackner and colleagues in the Journal of Urology reported that based on the available research during the past 25 years, CBT has the best evidence of effectiveness in the treatment of depression caused by chronic pelvic pain. (7) There is, unfortunately, limited scientific data about psychological treatments for depression and even less for the treatment of pain catastrophizing in men with chronic prostatitis. The limited research that has been done, however, points to psychotherapy, especially CBT, as being beneficial for treating depression in men with chronic prostatitis.

Antidepressant Medications

Much of the research done on the use of antidepressants for chronic prostatitis and chronic pelvic pain has focused primarily on treating pain rather than depression. The potential of the antidepressants studied to improve the symptoms of depression has been, in many cases, measured and evaluated as a secondary benefit. Therefore, we don't have a great deal of rigorous scientific research on the use of antidepressants to treat depression. The few studies that have been done, however, are promising.

A 2005 study by Lee and colleagues evaluated the serotonin-specific reuptake inhibitor (SSRI) antidepressant, Sertraline, as a treatment for the pain, urinary, sexual, and depression symptoms of chronic prostatitis during a 13-week study period. For depression symptoms, the study used the Hospital Anxiety & Depression (HAD) scale to measure the severity of depression. In addition to the improvements in the pain and urination symptoms, the study reported a significant decline in the depression severity score on the HAD scale. **(8)** One possible theory is that antidepressants work by lowering pain, which in turn, in a virtuous circle, reduces depression, and the lower depression helps reduce the pain. If this theory is accurate, the question becomes, do we need antidepressant drugs to create this virtuous cycle? Is it possible, for example, to use saw palmetto extract or pollen extract to create a similar vitreous cycle of reduced pain, improved depression, and reduced pain without using drugs with negative side effects? In other words, was the Sertraline in this study effective in improving depression

CHAPTER 10
Chronic Prostatitis and Depression

because it lowered pain, or did it work directly in improving depression and indirectly by lowering pain?

A 2017 Study by Zhang and colleagues with 126 participants divided into three groups compared two antidepressants, Duloxetine and Sertraline, and the alpha-blocker Doxazosin during a 6-month study. The study evaluated the impact on chronic prostatitis, pain, and depression symptoms using three separate scales. After 6 months, the researchers reported substantial improvements in the chronic prostatitis, pain, and depression symptoms in the Duloxetine group. Significant but less dramatic improvements were made in the Sertraline group, and relatively weak results were found in the Doxazosin group in all three symptom categories. **(9)** The study concluded that the antidepressant Duloxetine was particularly effective in treating depression, pain, and chronic prostatitis symptoms. The study, however, had limitations. The severity of the pain, depression, and chronic prostatitis symptoms of the participants in the study were mild to moderate, and the number of participants was small.

A Study by Xia and colleagues is an example of a study done using an antidepressant drug as a potential treatment for chronic prostatitis symptoms that did not directly analyze the impact on depression. In the 2011 study, 42 men diagnosed with chronic prostatitis were administered the SSRI antidepressant Fluoxetine for 12 weeks. The study reported significant improvements in pain and urinary symptoms. The researchers didn't directly measure the impact of the drug on depression, but they speculated it may have been effective, at least in part, by lowering depression. **(10)**

Most of the studies discussed above were primarily focused on treating the pain symptoms of chronic prostatitis. There was compelling evidence that many antidepressants are, in fact, successful in significantly reducing the pain symptoms of chronic prostatitis. And since pain is the primary underlying cause of severe depression, if an antidepressant can successfully treat pain, it can, in the process, improve the symptoms of severe depression. The theory is that antidepressants, in effect, work in two ways. Indirectly by improving the pain symptoms and directly by improving the depression symptoms. However, there is not enough evidence that anti-depressants are as effective as the three primary phytotherapies in the 360 Protocol for the treatment of pain discussed in Chapter 4.

A great deal more research is necessary on the benefits of anti-depressants in general, especially for men with more severe depression symptoms. While there isn't enough rigorous scientific research on antidepressants, they are, along with CBT, two treatment options that have demonstrated significant improvement in depression in men with chronic prostatitis. If you're struggling with chronic prostatitis and serious depression, it's important to recognize that there are scientifically proven treatments available for you. It's also critical to take immediate action and begin working with a mental health professional to treat your depression.

What follows is an outline of the role of relatively mild stress, anxiety, and depression in chronic prostatitis and what we can do to manage these symptoms in addition to working with a doctor or healthcare professional who specializes in treating more severe stress, anxiety, and depression. If you need professional help, the self-care steps discussed below should complement and enhance the professional treatment program you receive, but of course, always discuss any self-care measures you implement or plan to implement, such as exercise or supplements, with your doctor. Some of what is discussed below, such as meditation and exercise, may also overlap with the treatment program provided by a mental health professional. If you have mild stress and anxiety, you may be able

CHAPTER 10
Chronic Prostatitis and Depression

to manage them on your own using a combination of the self-care options discussed below.

The Management of Stress, Anxiety, and Mild Depression

There are many things you can do to help manage your stress, anxiety, and mild depression. The following are some important basic first steps:

1. Communication. Have a direct and honest discussion with every important person in your life. Tell them in blunt, direct language what you're living with every day. As men, we have a lifetime of socialization that encourages us to "be tough," "be strong," "to be a man..." and not be open about the difficulties and challenges, especially if it involves our emotions, psychological stress, or health issues related to our "private parts." One study found that 40% of men don't seek professional treatment for their chronic prostatitis. **(11)** But your spouse, adult children if you're older, other immediate family members, or close friends, doctors, etc., need to understand what you're living with, how you feel, and how it may impact your relationships and interactions with everyone important to you in your life. If the people closest to you don't clearly understand what you're living with, it can deepen your sense of social isolation and make it more difficult to respond to the many challenges of chronic prostatitis. Your family and friends can also play an important role in helping implement the diet and lifestyle changes in the protocol, but only if they understand what you're doing and why it's important.

2. Social Support. Building and maintaining what medical researchers call social support plays an important role in treating stress, anxiety, and depression and is often incorporated into psychotherapy treatment programs for depression in men with chronic prostatitis. You must make a conscious, consistent effort to reach out to your close family and friends to engage and communicate with them on a regular basis at a time when it can be more difficult to do so.

3. Hope. Don't give up hope. Even if you have struggled with this condition for years, there is reason for hope. There are scientifically proven treatments that do work in many cases. These treatments are not widely known or used in the US, but they have been proven in Europe and other parts of the world. There is, in short, reason to hope. One of the major goals of this book is to create awareness about the treatments that work and restore hope.

4. Action. Take action, control, and responsibility for treating your condition. Don't wait for others to figure out your condition and solve your problem. Reading this book, implementing the Prostatitis 360 Protocol, and starting the process of doing your research are important first steps. Taking action is, in other words, more than just scheduling yet another appointment with yet another urologist in a quest to find one that will finally have a cure for you. Taking action gives you greater control over the future course of treating your condition.

CHAPTER 10
Chronic Prostatitis and Depression

What follows is a review of the things you can do to help manage your stress and anxiety beyond the initial steps discussed above. They are not a cure for stress, anxiety, and depression; they are intended to help reduce and manage your symptoms on a day-to-day basis. They may also help to some extent with mild or even moderate depression in some cases. They often complement a treatment program developed by a mental health professional to treat your depression. It's important, however, to discuss any steps you take or plan to take to manage your stress and anxiety with the mental health professional who is treating your depression. The treatments and interventions discussed below have been included because they have substantial scientific evidence that they provide significant or meaningful benefits in the treatment of stress, anxiety, mild depression, and, in some cases, moderate depression or even more severe depression, especially when combined with CBT and antidepressants.

Exercise

Exercise, especially aerobic exercise may be one of the most important things you can do yourself to help manage your stress, anxiety, and mild depression. It also plays a role in helping with erectile dysfunction and reducing the inflammation associated with chronic prostatitis. Aerobic exercise is a key component of the lifestyle changes recommended in the Prostatitis 360 Protocol. If you have already begun implementing the protocol but have not yet reached the lifestyle stage of the protocol, implementing that stage of the protocol, including the aerobic exercise component, should also help with managing your stress, anxiety, and mild depression. The lifestyle chapter includes a detailed discussion of how to start and implement an aerobic exercise program for any level of aerobic exercise fitness and cardiovascular health. You can refer to the aerobic exercise section of the lifestyle chapter for additional information. While I discuss this in detail in the lifestyle chapter, it bears repeating here that if you're over 40, 50, or 60 and have lived a sedentary life in recent years—regardless of how physically fit you may have been in your 20s and 30s—it is absolutely critical that you start very slowly and consult with your primary care doctor, mental health professional (if you're being treated for depression), and cardiologist (if you have heart disease) before starting an aerobic exercise program. In short, there is compelling evidence that exercise provides significant benefits and should be incorporated into your plan to manage stress, anxiety, and mild depression.

There is some scientific evidence that exercise may be more effective than meditation programs, for example, in helping with anxiety, depression, pain, and quality of life. A meta-analysis of 47 studies and 3,320 participants done by Goyal and colleagues at Johns Hopkins University in 2014 found that exercise was more effective after 3 and 6 months than meditation programs. **(12)** The study found that meditation provided moderate benefits for anxiety, depression, and pain and low benefits for overall quality of life and was less effective than exercise. A more recent meta-analysis done by Singh and colleagues in 2023 involving 1039 trials and 128,119 participants concluded that "Physical activity should be a mainstay approach in the management of depression, anxiety, and psychological distress." **(13)** Studies also show that combining aerobic exercise and CBT or antidepressants is more effective than CBT or antidepressants alone. A meta-analysis done by Bourbeau and colleagues in 2020 analyzed 18 studies with 1686 participants and concluded that adding aerobic exercise to CBT significantly improves the symptoms of depression. The meta-analysis also showed that aerobic exercise was better than a combination of

CHAPTER 10
Chronic Prostatitis and Depression

aerobic and resistance training, that results improved with age, and that greater aerobic exercise intensity improved results.

There is compelling evidence that exercise provides a significant benefit and should be incorporated into your plan to manage your stress and depression. If you do only one thing to manage your stress, exercise may be the single best thing you can do. Ideally, you should, of course, combine several alternative and complementary treatments to manage your stress and depression. The effectiveness of different treatments varies from individual to individual, and the best strategy is to try several treatments to determine which treatment or combination treatments work best for you.

Meditation

There is a great deal of medical research done during the past 25 years that consistently shows that meditation is beneficial for treating stress, anxiety, and depression. A large-scale meta-analysis done during the past 15 years reports that meditation provides a moderate level of benefit in treating depression and the stress and anxiety that often lead to depression. There is a consensus among medical researchers who study depression that meditation should be part of an overall treatment program for many individuals suffering from depression. The Goyal study referenced above and a more recent meta-analysis done by Buric and colleagues in 2022, involving 51 studies and 7782 participants, concluded that meditation provides a "moderate" level of benefit in treating stress, anxiety, and depression. **(14)** These two large-scale meta-analyses, as well as similar recent studies, also report that there is a great deal of variation in who benefits and how much they benefit. Another important observation in many of these studies is that individuals suffering from higher levels of stress are more likely to see greater benefits from meditation.

Meditation is a broad term. There are several types of meditation, including Mindfulness-Based Therapy (MBT), Transcendental Meditation (TM), Acceptance and Commitment Therapy (ACT), Biofeedback, and others. Meta-analysis of these types of meditation reports similar results. A study of TM, for example, by Orme-Johnson and colleagues done in 2014 involving 16 studies and 1295 participants concluded that TM provides a moderate level of benefit and that individuals suffering from greater anxiety are likely to see greater benefit. **(15)** Which, if any, of these types of meditation will be available to you will depend on whether the healthcare professional you work with has integrated meditation as part of his or her practice and if your health insurance covers it. Most health insurance plans in the US don't cover meditation. You may have to go outside of your network if you have a PPO plan or do it at your own expense if you can afford it. You may be able to do some helpful basic relaxation techniques on your own, but proven meditation programs require professional training and guidance.

Yoga

Yoga as a treatment or intervention for stress, anxiety, and depression has been extensively studied during the past 25 years. The individual studies and the meta-analyses have consistently shown that yoga provides a significant or meaningful but moderate reduction in stress, anxiety, and mild depression. These studies conclude that there is enough evidence of the effectiveness of yoga to justify incorporating it as part of an overall treatment program for depression that incorporates CBT and/or antidepressants. A meta-analysis by Kramer and colleagues in 2013, for example, analyzed

CHAPTER 10
Chronic Prostatitis and Depression

12 RCTs with 619 participants and concluded that yoga significantly improves symptoms of depression. **(16)** A meta-analysis done by Atezaz and colleagues in 2019 analyzed exercise, meditation, yoga, and Tai chi studies. The meta-analysis of 11 yoga studies and systematic reviews reported that "systematic reviews and multiple individual studies conclude that yoga is an effective treatment for mild depression" but can only be recommended as an "adjunctive treatment with cognitive behavior therapy" and antidepressants for major anxiety disorders. The overall assessment of the study authors was that yoga, exercise, and meditation were comparable in terms of benefits and limitations in treating depression and major anxiety disorders, while the evidence for the benefits of Tai chi was mixed. **(17)** The study by Simon and colleagues done in 2021 with 226 male and female participants is particularly interesting. The 3-month study was designed to compare the effectiveness of kundalini yoga, CBT, and stress management education for treating depression. The study participants were divided into three groups and assigned one of the treatments. After three months, 71% of the CBT group reported a significant improvement compared to 54% for the yoga group and no meaningful improvement in the stress education group. The study authors concluded that while yoga was not as effective as CBT, it can be a valuable complementary or adjunctive intervention alongside CBT and antidepressant treatment plans. **(18)**

Yoga is another treatment or intervention option available to you alongside exercise and meditation for the management of stress, anxiety, and depression. There are several types of yoga, including hatha, kundalini, isha, and raja yoga, among others. The most common style of yoga practiced in the US is hatha yoga. It's the style of yoga that is widely recommended and researched in the US for the treatment of stress, anxiety, and depression. Yoga is not covered by health insurance in the US. The best way to learn yoga is to take a weekly class for 8 to 12 weeks. Studies show that the benefits of yoga fade when it's discontinued. The best way to use yoga to manage your stress and depression is to make it part of your daily routine.

Massage Therapy

Massage therapy does not have the same level of scientific evidence to support its effectiveness as the other treatments we've discussed so far. But there is enough evidence that it should be one of the options you consider. A meta-analysis by Hou and colleagues, conducted in 2010, analyzed 17 studies with 786 participants and reported that 'All the trials showed a positive effect of massage therapy on depressed individuals **(19)**. A particularly interesting study was done by Poland and colleagues in 2013. In the study, 37 participants diagnosed with depression were given Swedish massages twice a week for one hour for 8 weeks. The researchers used the Hamilton Depression Rating Scale (HAM-D) to measure progress and outcomes. Many of the participants began to see improvement by week 4 and significant improvements by weeks 6 to 8. The participants reported, on average, a 43.3% reduction in depression based on the HAM-D depression scale, and just over 50% of the participants had at least a 50% or greater reduction in depression. The study also compared participants who were treated with massage therapy alone and those who were treated with a combination of massage therapy and antidepressants. The participants treated with massage therapy alone had a 41% improvement in depression, and those who received the combination treatment had a 47% improvement. **(20)** This is an example of how combining conventional medical treatment for depression, such as CBT and antidepressants, with complementary and alternative medicine (CAM) can be beneficial for treating depression.

Massage therapy has several advantages compared to other alternative treatments. It is widely available in the US, is relatively inexpensive, does not require training, and can be done weekly rather than daily. Researchers have not established an optimal frequency and duration for massage therapy. Some studies show that one weekly 45-minute massage is enough to be effective. One strategy may be to start with two weekly 60-minute massage sessions and, after six to eight weeks, reduce it to one weekly 45-minute massage, as long as it proves to be effective. Massage therapy is not covered by health insurance in the US. We have no data on the use of massage therapy by psychiatrists and other mental health professionals as a complementary treatment. We have some limited data on the use of massage therapy as an alternative treatment by individuals with depression. One survey, for example, reported that 54% of women use massage therapy to help treat depression. **(21)**

Lifestyle Changes

There are several lifestyle factors that have an impact on the prevention and treatment of stress, anxiety, and depression. The three most common factors in studies of the role of lifestyle in preventing and treating depression are a healthy diet, regular exercise, and quality sleep. A recent large-scale population study of the prevention of depression done by Zhao and colleagues in 2023 reported that seven lifestyle factors played a particularly important role in preventing depression. The top four ranked by the percentage they reduce depression risk were: Quality sleep 22%, never smoking 20%, frequent social interaction 18%, and regular exercise 14%. The other three were avoiding sedentary behavior 13%, moderate alcohol consumption 11%, and healthy diet 6%. The study found that participants who had followed five or more of these factors were 57% less likely to develop depression. **(22)** In terms of treating depression, most studies show that the top three lifestyle factors that reduce depression are sleep quality, regular exercise, and diet. A study by Aguilar-Latorre and colleagues done in 2022 concluded that a healthy diet, regular exercise, and good sleep quality significantly improved depression symptoms. **(23)** A 2021 meta-analysis by Wang and colleagues, which analyzed 50 studies with 8,479 participants, concluded that lifestyle changes provided a significant but small benefit in reducing the symptoms of depression but were not effective for severe depression. **(24)** Regular exercise, as discussed above, has been extensively studied as a standalone treatment and has proven to be effective in managing symptoms of stress and reducing depression.

Many of the most important lifestyle changes recommended for preventing and treating depression are an integral part of the Prostatitis 360 Protocol for treating chronic prostatitis, including a healthy diet, avoiding alcohol, improving the quality of sleep, and regular aerobic exercise. If you have already begun to implement the diet and lifestyle parts of the protocol, they can help prevent depression, and if you have depression, they can help treat it. These diet and lifestyle changes are important for preventing the inflammation that plays a role in causing chronic prostatitis, as well as preventing and treating depression.

Supplements

The research done during the past 25 years on the use of supplements to treat depression has demonstrated that some supplements can play a role in the treatment of mild and moderate depression and even, in some cases, more serious depression. This form of depression is also known as clinical depression or major depressive disorder. In the case of serious depression, the role of supplements is primarily as an add-on or complementary treatment for antidepressant drugs. However, for those individuals who don't respond to antidepressant drugs or who cannot tolerate the side effects of these drugs, supplements can be an alternative. In the case of mild to moderate depression that does not warrant the use of antidepressant drugs, there are also some supplements that have been proven to be effective for treating moderate depression. You should only consider supplements as a treatment option after discussing them with your doctor and only with his or her approval. Some doctors may already be using supplements. But in many cases, it may be up to you to make the case for the use of supplements based on scientific research about effectiveness and the fact that supplements have important advantages compared to prescription drugs. The most important advantage for you to consider and discuss with your doctor is the fact that supplements rarely have any significant side effects. On the other hand, if you're taking any prescription drugs, some supplements can interact with them. Therefore, it's very important to discuss the use of supplements with your doctors prior to starting any supplement if you are taking prescription drugs. While the case for the use of some supplements for treating moderate depression and serious depression has substantial scientific evidence.

The role of supplements in the treatment of stress and mild anxiety is less clear. In most cases, the supplements that are promoted as helping with stress and anxiety lack the kind of extensive, rigorous scientific research that would be required to make any informed judgments about their effectiveness.

Supplements Combined with Anti-Depression Drugs for Serious Depression

The primary treatment for serious depression, what the medical profession calls the first line of treatment, is, first and foremost, the use of psychotherapy and antidepressant drugs. If these treatments prove to be ineffective or antidepressant drugs involve unacceptably serious side effects, supplements can be a potential alternative treatment or a complementary treatment for antidepressant drugs. It may be possible, for example, in the case of an antidepressant drug that is effective but has serious side effects, to add a supplement that enhances the effectiveness of the drug and lowers the dosage, which reduces the undesirable side effects. What follows is a discussion of 3 supplements with scientific research that provides evidence that when they are combined with antidepressants, they enhance the effectiveness of those drugs.

Probiotics

There is a great deal of interest in the use of probiotics in the treatment of depression. Probiotics have been extensively studied both as stand-alone treatments for depression and in combination with antidepressant drugs. There have been at least 6 meta-analyses done during the past 10 years alone involving over 100 RCT studies.

CHAPTER 10
Chronic Prostatitis and Depression

A meta-analysis of the studies done between 2014 and 2023 by Merkouris and colleagues selected 31 high-quality meta-analyses and individual RCT studies of patients taking antidepressants. The studies included both patients with mild to moderate depression and those with serious depression or major depressive disorder (MDD). Almost all the studies were based on a combination of multiple probiotic strains. Most of the studies in this analysis reported that adding probiotics to antidepressant treatment significantly improved the symptoms of depression. **(25)** A meta-analysis by Zhang and colleagues, done in 2023, involving 13 studies with 786 participants, analyzed individuals with moderate depression who were not taking antidepressants. The researchers reported that the probiotic treatment resulted in a significant improvement in the symptoms of depression in individuals with moderate depression. **(26)** Several recent individual studies have also reported that probiotics combined with antidepressant drugs enhance the effectiveness of those drugs. A study by Bistas and colleagues, done in 2023, involved 81 patients with moderate to serious depression taking antidepressants. After eight weeks, the researchers reported that there was a significant decrease in depression scores using the Beck's Depression Inventory (BDI) index. The BDI index is one of the commonly used measures of depression. Studies also show that probiotics can be effective in cases where antidepressants provide little or moderate benefit. A 2023 study by Nikolova and colleagues involved 50 participants with major depressive disorder taking antidepressants with partial or limited benefit. After eight weeks, 84% of the individuals who added antibiotics to their existing antidepressant treatments reported improvement, including 52% who reported "much improved" or "very much improved" results. Only 16% reported no improvement. **(27)** There's even some preliminary evidence that probiotics may be effective in cases where conventional medical treatment, such as antidepressants, does not work. A study done by Miyaoka and colleagues in 2018 involved 40 participants with major depressive disorder or serious depression who had Treatment-Resistant Depression (TRD). Unlike almost all studies that use multiple strains of probiotics, this study used a single strain of probiotics called Clostridium butyricum. The study found that "70% of the participants responded after eight weeks and 35% reported remission". This is a substantial improvement for individuals with major depressive disorder who have TRD depression. However, it's important to caution that this one small study is not enough. A great deal more research will have to be done before we can draw any meaningful conclusions about the use of this strain of probiotics for major depressive disorder and TRD. **(28)** Despite being very promising, this study has not been replicated. Probiotics research has been limited. While many studies have been done during the past 25 years, most of them are short-term. A typical study lasts about 8 weeks. We don't have enough data about long-term treatment benefits.

There is no consensus about which probiotic strains should be used for treating depression. The most common probiotic strains used in depression studies are in the **Lactobacillus and Bifidobacterium probiotic groups, with a minimum dose of 10 CFU.** Despite the wide variety of probiotic strains used in studies, most of those studies report that probiotics provide a significant benefit in treating depression. Probiotics have some important advantages compared to antidepressant drugs, which can involve serious side effects. Studies show that the side effects of probiotics for treating depression are rare and minor. Potential drug interactions include antibiotic and antifungal prescription drugs. If you're taking any prescription drugs, you should always discuss the use of probiotics

CHAPTER 10
Chronic Prostatitis and Depression

or any other supplement with your doctor prior to starting probiotics. Despite some of the limitations of probiotics, there is, on balance, enough extensive and rigorous scientific research to make a compelling case for probiotics as a stand-alone treatment and as a treatment combined with antidepressants for both moderate and serious depression. If you're currently taking antidepressants, you should discuss the use of probiotics with your doctor prior to starting them. Most studies typically take four weeks of probiotic treatment to see initial results and eight weeks for significant improvement.

Zinc

A meta-analysis and individual studies have been done to research the effectiveness of zinc combined with antidepressant drugs to treat serious or major depressive disorder (MDD) during the past 25 years. In most cases, these studies combined 25 mg of Zinc with the SSRI class of antidepressant drugs, and the patients in the studies were clinically diagnosed with serious depression. A meta-analysis done by Da Silva and colleagues in 2020 analyzed 5 studies that combined 25mg of zinc and SSRIs in studies that ranged from 2 to 6 months. The researchers reported that zinc combined with antidepressants was significantly more effective than antidepressants alone. **(29)** An earlier similar meta-analysis done in 2016 by Schefft and colleagues involving 4 studies reported similar results. A study done by Ranjbar and colleagues in 2013 involved 44 patients diagnosed with major depressive disorder (MDD) who were being treated with SSRIs. The study participants were divided into two groups: one group continued with SSRI treatments alone, and the other group combined their SSRI treatment with 25 milligrams of zinc. The Beck Depression Inventory (BDI) was used to measure the level of depression. The study participants had similar scores at the start of the study. At the end of the three-month study, the BDI scores of the group that combined zinc and SSRIs were significantly lower compared to the SSRI group. The researchers concluded that adding 25 mg of zinc can significantly improve the symptoms of patients currently being treated with SSRIs alone. **(30)**

While the research that has been done so far on the use of zinc in combination with SSRIs to treat serious depression is promising, a great deal more research will have to be done before it can be compared to probiotics. The level of evidence supporting probiotics as a standalone treatment and a combination treatment with SSRIs is vastly superior. If, however, adding probiotics to antidepressant treatment is not effective, zinc can be another option for you to discuss with your doctor if you're currently being treated with antidepressants. Zinc is a secondary option to consider if probiotics are not effective. There is also no evidence, unlike probiotics, that zinc is effective as a standalone treatment for serious depression. Therefore, unlike probiotics, zinc is not an option for individuals with serious depression who have not responded to antidepressant drug treatment. Zinc may be a treatment option for mild depression. We discuss zinc along with several other potential treatments for mild depression in a section later in this chapter that is focused on supplements for treating mild depression.

Omega-3

Omega is another option for serious depression in combination with antidepressant drugs. There is not enough evidence that omega-3 is effective as a standalone treatment for serious depression. The studies that have been done show weak results. As in the case of zinc, the evidence supporting omega-3 as a treatment for serious depression combined with antidepressants is not as compelling as that for probiotics. Three meta-analyses done by Mocking and colleagues with 13 studies, Schefft and colleagues with 4 studies, and Sarris and colleagues with four studies all reported that adding 1000 to 2000 mg of omega-3 EPA with a 3:1 ratio of EPA to DHA significantly improved the symptoms of serious depression in patients being treated with antidepressants. While these results are promising, the quality and quantity of evidence for probiotics is much stronger. Until there is further extensive research, Omega 3 is a secondary or backup option to discuss with your doctor in cases where combining omega-3 and antidepressants is not effective. Studies of omega-3 combinations with antidepressants show that side effects are rare and minor. If you are taking any prescription drugs, as in the case of all supplements, you should check with your doctor before you take Omega-3. There is also evidence that Omega 3 is effective as a treatment for mild to moderate depression when combined with antidepressants. We will discuss supplements combined with antidepressants for mild to moderate depression below. There are several other supplements that have been researched as complementary treatments for serious depression. However, there is a lack of rigorous scientific evidence as to their effectiveness either because there are too few studies, which is the case with most of them, or the studies that have been done have mixed results.

Supplements Combined with Antidepressants for Mild to Moderate

There are three supplements, Omega-3, folate, and probiotics, with evidence that when they are combined with antidepressants, they enhance the effectiveness of those drugs in the treatment of mild to moderate depression. Zinc is not included because while there is evidence that it's effective for serious depression, there is little scientific data on its use to treat mild to moderate depression. It's plausible that if zinc is effective in treating serious depression, it may also help with mild and moderate depression, but there is a lack of scientific evidence.

Omega-3

A meta-analysis done by Sarris and colleagues in 2016 analyzed eight studies of patients clinically diagnosed with moderate depression and taking antidepressants. The meta-analysis showed that adding omega-3 to the existing antidepressant treatment significantly improved depression symptoms. A study done by Medhi and colleagues in 2023 involved 165 patients with mild to moderate depression. In the study, the patients were divided into three groups: patients who took SSRIs alone, patients who took omega-3 alone, and those who took a combination of SSRIs and omega-3. The study used 500 milligrams of omega-3 and one of three different SSRIs, including Escitalopram 10mg, Sertraline 100mg, and Fluoxetine 20mg. All the study participants started the study at the same level of depression. At the end of the three-month study, the patients who took Omega 3 combined with one of the 3 SSRIs had significantly better improvements in depression symptoms than either the participants who only took SSRIs or Omeaga-3 alone. The combination treatment was more effective than the antidepressant treatment alone. All three antidepressants work equally well in combination with omega-3. **(31)** There is enough rigorous scientific research to warrant considering Omega-3 for mild to moderate depression.

Folic Acid

A meta-analysis done by Gao and colleagues in 2024 analyzed 14 RCT studies with 1,046 participants diagnosed with depression and treated with prescription antidepressants. The meta-analysis concluded that folic acid "significantly relieved depression" symptoms when combined with antidepressants. **(32)** On average, the studies were ten weeks long. The dosage used in the studies ranged from 500 mcg of folic acid to 15 mg of methyl folate. Folic acid is another term for folate, and methyl folate is believed to be a more bioavailable form of folate and is preferred by some doctors. Please note that 15 milligrams of methyl folate is extremely high and should only be taken under strict medical supervision. Most of the studies used a much lower dosage of 500mcg to 1500mcg. One theory holds that individuals who have depression are more likely to be deficient in folic acid, which may explain why folic acid is effective in treating depression when combined with antidepressants. However, studies have produced mixed results, with some showing that individuals with normal levels of folic acid also benefit from adding folic acid to antidepressants. An earlier meta-analysis done in 2016 by Sarris and colleagues analyzed 9 studies of participants who added folic acid to their existing SSRI treatment program. The researchers in this meta-analysis also reported that adding folic acid significantly enhanced SSRI treatment outcomes. A 52-week study done by Almeida and colleagues in 2014 is particularly interesting because it was a long-term study focused on patients over 50. The study found that adding 2mg of folic acid, 500mcg of B-12, and 25mg of B6 to the SSRI Citalopram (20-40mg) significantly improved depression symptoms after 52 weeks compared to Citalopram alone. It's important to note that the study found no improvement after 12 weeks and a small improvement after 26 weeks. In this study, it took 52 weeks to see a significant improvement among the participants in the supplement group. Most studies of folic acid show improvements after 8 to 12 weeks. This suggests that it may take much longer for older individuals over 50 to see significant benefits from adding folic acid, B12, and B6 to antidepressants. This is important in the case of chronic prostatitis because 50% of the men with chronic prostatitis are over 50. **(33)**

Probiotics

The discussion of probiotics for the treatment of serious depression above in the section on serious depression also includes important studies of probiotics combined with antidepressants to treat moderate depression. The meta-analyses done by Merkouris and Colleagues in 2023 and Bistas and colleagues in 2023 referenced above both analyzed the use of probiotics with antidepressants for moderate depression and concluded that probiotics provide significant improvement in mild and moderate depression.

As in the case of the use of supplements for serious depression, there are a number of supplements that have been studied in conjunction with antidepressants for the treatment of mild and moderate depression. However, there is a lack of rigorous scientific evidence as to their effectiveness, either because there are too few studies, which is the case with most of them, or the studies that have been done have mixed results, or the studies done were too small and of poor quality.

Stand-alone treatments for mild stress, anxiety, and depression

An Internet search for treatments for mild stress, anxiety, and depression symptoms results in a long list of purported treatments and supplements that make largely unsubstantiated claims about helping improve the symptoms of stress and anxiety. Supplement companies promote a wide range of supplements with various claims about helping with stress and anxiety. But in most cases, there was very little or no rigorous scientific research to back up those claims.

St. John's Wort

St. John's Wort, or SJW, is one of the few supplements with a long history of use and extensive, rigorous scientific research. SJW has been used in Europe, especially in Germany, for over 100 years by mental health professionals to treat stress, anxiety, and mild to moderate depression. In Germany, it is regarded as a prescription medication that is often prescribed by doctors. It is, however, also available over the counter without a prescription. During the past 50 years, there have been hundreds of studies involving thousands of participants, many of them done in Germany. The focus here is on the research done during the past 25 years.

The largest meta-analyses conducted over the past 25 years, including, for example, 27 studies analyzed by Benitez and colleagues between 2011 and 2021, have shown significant findings. **(34)**, 35 studies involving 6993 participants analyzed by Apaydin and colleagues and 27 studies with 3126 participants analyzed by Cui and colleagues have, in most cases, come to a remarkably consistent conclusion about the role of SJW in treating depression. The conclusions include: SJW is significantly better than placebo as a stand-alone treatment for mild depression. In many cases, it can be comparable in terms of the level of effectiveness to antidepressant drugs in treating moderate depression but without the serious side effects that many patients experience with antidepressant drugs.

SJW is not an effective treatment for serious depression, either stand-alone or in combination with antidepressant drugs. Most studies of SJW use 900 milligrams a day divided into three 300-milligram doses taken during the day.

SJW has fewer side effects in general and fewer serious side effects compared to antidepressant drugs based on data from thousands of individuals taking SJW studied during the past 25 years. However, it's very important to caution that SJW has several potentially serious drug interactions. In Germany, where it's widely prescribed by doctors, it is carefully monitored and screened for potential drug interactions. Most of the studies done during the past 25 years have been done in Germany, and therefore, most of the data on side effects and drug interactions has come from Germany. In the US, on the other hand, unless a doctor or psychiatrist has experience with the use of SJW for the treatment of depression, it is largely up to the individual patient to carefully review the list of potential drug interactions against any prescription drugs he or she is taking and discuss it with their doctors. It is estimated that SJW has potential drug interactions with 50% of prescription drugs. This is the level of individual patient responsibility that some individuals suffering from mild to moderate depression may not be comfortable with. In the face of the caution and safety concerns of SJW, it may not be a viable option for many individuals with mild to moderate depression who are taking prescription medications.

L-Methyl Folate

L-methyl folate is a specific form of folic acid that is proven in several studies to be effective in treating depression stand-alone as well as combined with SSRIs. L-methyl folate, unlike St John's Wort, can be combined with SSSIs to treat more serious depression. A study by Shelton and colleagues of 502 patients who added 15 mg of Deplin (a prescription form of L-Methyl Folate) with their existing SSRI drug treatments and 52 patients who took Deplin stand-alone reported significant improvement. After 95 days, 67.9% of the patients saw an average 58.2% improvement in their depression symptoms, and 45.7% achieved remission. (.) Deplin is sold by prescription, but it's labeled as a "medical food" and is not a drug. There are no scientific studies of over-the-counter versions of L-methyl folate. **(35)** Despite the lack of clear scientific evidence, over-the-counter L-Methylfolate is widely sold and used as a treatment for depression.

SAMe

SAMe is an over-the-counter supplement that has generally proven to be effective and provides moderate to significant improvement in mild to moderate depression symptoms. A 2020 meta-analysis of 11 studies involving 1,011 participants who took SAMe as a standalone and as an add-on therapy for prescription depression medications showed a significant improvement in symptoms as a standalone treatment and as a combination treatment. The dosage ranged from 200 milligrams to 3,200 milligrams, with the typical dosage of 1600 milligrams. Side effects were rare, mild, and transient. **(36)** Studies have shown that increasing the dosage from 1600 milligrams to 3200 milligrams results in improved benefits.

Saffron

Saffron is an herb that is available as an over-the-counter supplement in pill form. It has proven to be effective in several studies in treating stress and anxiety, as well as moderate depression. A meta-analysis of 9 studies by Toth et al. involving participants with moderate subclinical depression showed that taking saffron significantly reduced the symptoms of depression. The typical dosage in these studies was 15 mg 2x/day for a total of 30 mg a day. **(37)** Several studies of saffron for anxiety, stress, and moderate (subclinical) depression have shown similar results in treating these conditions using the same dosage.

There are supplements that have been studied for mild to moderate depression, anxiety, and stress, including EPA /DPA Fish Oil, 5HTP, and vitamin B12. However, to date, these studies have been limited and inconclusive. Research on 5HTP has been promising, but there are concerns about potential serious side effects. There are several vitamins and minerals believed to help with mild depression and anxiety, including B complex vitamins, vitamin D, and magnesium.

If you have mild or moderate depression and you're not able to take SJW due to potential drug interactions, and in the case of moderate depression, you find that antidepressant drugs involve too many serious side effects, the list above can be a starting point for doing additional research to determine if they can help with your mild or moderate depression.

There is a great deal of variation in individual responses to depression treatments. In the case of antidepressant drugs, approximately one out of three individuals is not helped, or the side effects are so serious that they choose to discontinue treatment. This varies a great deal by age, sex, presence of other serious medical conditions, and other variables and can range from approximately 20% to 40%. There are also several different kinds of antidepressant drugs, and in many cases, it's a process of trial and error to determine which works best for a given individual. The same, of course, is true for supplements for stress, anxiety, and various levels of depression. In either case, it's a trial-and-error process.

CHAPTER 10
Chronic Prostatitis and Depression

A Holistic Strategy

For most men with chronic prostatitis, their depression is the result of the chronic pain caused by chronic prostatitis, and therefore, the most important way to treat depression is to implement the Chronic Prostatitis 360 Protocol to dramatically reduce or eliminate the chronic pain that is the underlying cause of the depression. The roadmap to treating depression in men with chronic prostatitis is to use a holistic strategy that integrates:

1. Eliminating or dramatically reducing the chronic pain of chronic prostatitis by implementing the Chronic Prostatitis 360 Protocol.
2. Work with a mental health professional to treat your depression in the meantime.
3. Integrating complementary treatments and lifestyle changes as part of the overall treatment program.

If you're a man struggling with chronic prostatitis and depression, especially serious depression, the cornerstone of implementing this strategy is to immediately begin working with a mental health professional, typically a psychiatrist, to treat your depression. If you have not fully implemented the protocol or it's still early in the process of implementation, you should continue to work on implementing and maintaining the protocol while you work with your doctor to treat your depression.

Part IV
Going Forward

CHAPTER 11
The Future of the Chronic Prostatitis 360 Protocol

If you are a man struggling with chronic prostatitis and you just finished reading the book, you have confirmed in Chapter 1 that it is likely you have the condition, and you have begun to implement the protocol. It may be too early to contemplate the future of the protocol. I certainly understand that your focus right now is, as it should be, on implementing the protocol and achieving a dramatic reduction in the severity of your chronic prostatitis symptoms. If not, a complete cure or something approaching a 90% reduction in the severity of your symptoms should be your focus and goal at this stage. However, once you fully implement the protocol and see a dramatic, life-changing improvement in your severe chronic prostatitis symptoms, you can do a great deal to help other men attain their goal of a life-changing, dramatic improvement in their symptoms. I invite you to return once you have fully implemented the protocol to read this final chapter and join me in my mission to help every man in the US who is struggling with chronic prostatitis.

There are approximately 5 million men in the US who have chronic prostatitis ranging in age from 25 to 85 and beyond. **(1)** the goal of reaching and helping that many men is an enormous series of challenges and obstacles. There are four potential models for reaching such a large group of individuals with chronic prostatitis. These models are not mutually exclusive. In fact, the best strategy is to combine and integrate these models into a single strategy. However, it is helpful to analyze and understand each one as a standalone model.

1. The Direct Model: Directly Reaching & Educating Chronic Prostatitis Patients

In the direct model, we use a wide range of media, including books, articles, social media, YouTube, public speaking, radio, and television, to reach individuals struggling with chronic prostatitis directly. This book, the Chronic Prostatitis 360 Protocol website, blog, social media presence, and many other direct ways to reach men with chronic prostatitis are the starting point and foundation for implementing this and the other strategies. Directly reaching, informing, and educating 5 million men between the ages of 25 and 85 is an enormous undertaking. Pharmaceutical companies and consumer product companies spend 10s of millions of dollars on advertising to reach target audiences that large. The challenges of directly reaching a significant segment of these 5 million men in the short to medium term are substantial.

CHAPTER 11
The Future of the Chronic Prostatitis 360 Protocol

2. The Medical Establishment Model

The second model uses the medical establishment to reach patients treated by primary care doctors and doctors who specialize in treating a particular medical condition. This path usually involves doing extensive, rigorous medical research that is published in peer-reviewed medical journals, writing both books and articles geared for medical professionals as well as popular books geared for patients, and gaining recognition and acceptance by the medical establishment, including doctors, medical societies, medical journals, government health agencies, and health insurance companies among others. This is a largely indirect approach. First, you reach the doctors who, in turn, provide medical care with a new treatment approach to their patients. This is how Dr Ornish established the Ornish treatment program for heart disease as a credible treatment for many types of heart disease in the 1990s. The Ornish program gained wide and broad acceptance by doctors and the entire medical establishment in the US. He did extensive medical research in the 1980s and the 1990s published the results in highly respected peer-reviewed medical journals, and wrote successful best-selling books for the general reading public.

The Ornish program has become widely known and respected during the past 25 years by cardiologists, the heart disease medical establishment, and heart disease patients. It is a highly successful example of the large-scale acceptance by the medical community and by patients of a diet, supplement, lifestyle, and exercise treatment program for a major medical condition. What is less clear and is an open question is whether it has led to the wide-scale adoption or use of the Ornish program by cardiologists, the healthcare establishment, and patients. In other words, how many cardiologists have integrated the Ornish Program into their practice and are using it on a regular basis, and how many heart patients who could benefit from it are using it? One of the key insights or lessons learned from the Ornish program during the past 30 years is that cardiologists are not the best vehicle for implementing the Ornish Program. They can and should play an important role in educating their patients about the Ornish program. However, they do not have the time, resources, and skill set to train their patients to implement the Ornish program or find a way to be paid for it. Cardiologists do not have the training and experience as instructors, dietitians, exercise or meditation specialists to provide the necessary training effectively. What was needed was a way to provide the necessary training to patients, to find a way for healthcare providers to generate revenue to provide the training, and a way for patients to pay for the training. Doctor Ornish developed a 10-week certified training program offered by hospitals and clinics, which is paid for by Medicare and private health insurance.

3. Direct Training Model: Expanding Access to Ornish Program Training

After gaining wide acceptance for the Ornish program among cardiologists and the larger medical establishment, Dr Ornish, in recent years, created two new ways to expand access to the Ornish program. The first involves the creation of Ornish program-certified treatment centers in cooperation with hospitals and clinics around the country. Many heart patients need in-person step-by-step coaching, training, and motivational support to implement the rigorous Ornish diet, exercise, lifestyle, and supplement treatment program. Reading a book with detailed instructions on implementing the program is not enough for these patients. The cost

CHAPTER 11
The Future of the Chronic Prostatitis 360 Protocol

of the program offered at these certified treatment centers varies but is approximately $10,000. Medicare and many health insurance companies provide reimbursement for the program. This has allowed healthcare providers like hospitals a way to generate the revenue they need to offer the Ornish program. In the process, Dr Ornish created a model for hospitals and clinics to provide a diet and lifestyle treatment program to patients by charging a fee for a 10-week, on-site training program. This Model can be used for chronic prostatitis patients who need on-site, in-person coaching, training, and motivational support to implement the chronic prostatitis 360 protocol successfully.

However, once you have a $10,000 treatment program, you also need a way for patients to pay for that program. Most patients need private health insurance and Medicare reimbursement to pay for a $10,000 treatment. Dr Ornish spent 16 years working with Medicare to approve reimbursement for the Ornish program offered by hospitals and clinics. In 2010, Medicare approved reimbursement for the Ornish Program under Medicare Part B. Since then, a growing list of private health insurance companies have agreed to provide reimbursement for the Ornish Program. This is an important precedent for Medicare and private health insurance coverage for a diet and lifestyle treatment program such as the Chronic Prostatitis 360 protocol.

The other way Dr Ornish expanded access to the Ornish program was by creating an online nine-week program of live instructional classes. This online program is approximately $7,000 to $10,000. Some health insurance companies have begun to provide reimbursement for the program. This further expands access to the Ornish Program to anyone with Internet access anywhere in the US or around the world if they can afford the cost of the program or if it's covered by their health insurance company.

The Ornish in-person and online training programs are a model for how patients can successfully implement a diet, supplement, exercise, and lifestyle treatment program that requires very demanding and difficult diet and lifestyle changes. The Ornish program demands that men and women, predominantly in their 50s and beyond, adopt a vegetarian diet, stop caffeine, and eliminate or strictly limit alcohol. These diet changes alone represent a major challenge for anyone in their 50s or older who has spent decades, in many cases, eating the traditional American diet. A 10-week program of in-person small group classes that meet twice a week can provide the instruction and training and, perhaps more importantly, the motivational and peer group support necessary to implement and sustain difficult diet and lifestyle changes.

There are important advantages and disadvantages to online and in-person classes. The online classes provide near-universal access to the program throughout the US. However, the in-person programs have important advantages in that in-person classes offer an element of motivational and peer group support that is difficult to replicate in online classes. It is also easier to obtain health insurance reimbursement for in-person classes. Therefore, in the major metropolitan areas in the US where in-person classes are more widely available, they offer important advantages compared to online classes.

4. The UPOINT System

I briefly discussed the UPOINT System in Chapter 2. It would have to evolve a great deal to be a potential platform for the adoption of the Prostatitis 360 protocol. As it stands today, it is only a theoretical model or platform for bringing the Prostatitis 360 Protocol into the mainstream conventional U.S. healthcare system. In concept, it is

CHAPTER 11
The Future of the Chronic Prostatitis 360 Protocol

very similar to the Prostatitis 360 Protocol in that it recognizes that chronic prostatitis is caused by a wide range of different contributing factors or what medical researchers call a multifactorial disease and that what is needed is a multimodal treatment customized for each individual. Multimodal means drawing on a wide range of treatment types from many categories of treatment, just like the prostatitis 360 protocol. In other words, both the Prostatitis 360 Protocol and the UPOINT System recognize that chronic prostatitis is a multifactorial condition that can only be treated with a multimodal treatment program.

However, today, the UPOINT System has too many limitations. It is widely used by chronic prostatitis researchers in the US and around the world, but most practicing urologists in the US are not familiar with the system and don't use it. Today, it is almost entirely limited to conventional medical treatments that have proven to be largely ineffective in treating chronic prostatitis. There is no role for diet, supplements, or lifestyle changes in the current UPOINT System. When it was first introduced by two of the world's most prominent chronic prostatitis researchers in the early 2000s, it included quercetin and flower pollen among the treatment options, but in recent years, they have been either removed or de-emphasized. It requires a battery of tests that, while ideal, are highly unlikely to be covered by HMO and PPO health insurance in the foreseeable future. If, in the future, it became widely known, accepted, and used by urologists and the mainstream health care system and if it incorporated the elements of the chronic prostatitis 360 protocol, it could be a vehicle or platform for the adoption of the Prostatitis 360 Protocol by the mainstream health care system in the US. I believe it is highly unlikely in the foreseeable future that the UPOINT System will be widely adopted and that it will integrate the Prostatitis 360 Protocol among its treatment options.

The Ornish Model as a Model for the Prostatitis 360 Protocol

Dr. Ornish and his work with the Ornish Program over the past 40 years provide important insights and lessons learned that are valuable for the Prostatitis 360 protocol. These insights include:

1. A book, however detailed, is not enough for some patients to successfully implement a rigorous diet and lifestyle program.
2. Many patients need extensive in-person instruction and training, along with motivational and peer group support, to successfully implement and sustain a rigorous diet and lifestyle program.
3. Doctors in individual private practice, such as cardiologists and urologists, don't have the background training and experience to train their patients on the implementation of rigorous diet and lifestyle programs.
4. Healthcare providers need a way to generate revenue to provide in-depth, in-person training for patients who need a rigorous diet and lifestyle program.
5. Most patients need Medicare or private health insurance reimbursement to pay for the program.

These insights have important implications for the future of the Prostatitis 360 Protocol. Once the protocol is extensively studied and proven in rigorous scientific studies, widely known among chronic prostatitis patients, and widely accepted by urologists and the urology establishment, it will have to follow a similar evolution

CHAPTER 11
The Future of the Chronic Prostatitis 360 Protocol

to the Ornish Program. That means a comparable 10-week certified on-site training program offered by hospitals and clinics that are paid for by private health insurance or Medicare for patients who need in-person training with motivational and peer group support.

The Ornish program is the best model and road map we have for the wide-scale adoption of a diet, supplement, and lifestyle treatment similar to the Prostatitis 360 Protocol for a major medical condition in the US with a large population of patients. To successfully implement this model, the Prostatitis 360 Protocol will have to follow a similar roadmap of extensive, rigorous scientific research, publication in major medical journals, and gradual acceptance by the medical establishment, including the urological medical establishment, as well as informing and educating the chronic prostatitis patient community and offering individualized help with training, motivation and group support to implement the Prostatitis 360 Protocol. We will also need to follow a similar model of creating certified training programs to help patients implement the program, which will permit hospitals and clinics to generate revenue to offer the program, and that will require the time and effort necessary to lobby Medicare and private health insurance to provide reimbursement for the cost of the training program. As in the case of the Ornish program, this will require a great deal of time, effort, and resources, including substantial financial resources, starting with substantial funding for extensive, rigorous scientific research.

I believe we will need to establish a nonprofit foundation to raise money to fund research on the Chronic Prostatitis 360 Protocol and develop and execute the comprehensive strategy to promote the wide-scale adoption of the Prostatitis 360 Protocol in the US based on the Ornish model. The mission of helping 5 million American men with chronic prostatitis will require vision, strategy, and a team of individuals with a wide range of talents and a sense of mission to shape and execute the strategy. If you are reading this book and you have any experience or expertise or you know somebody who does in areas such as conventional or holistic medicine, medical research, fundraising, grant writing, nonprofit leadership, or management, there is an opportunity to get involved in supporting this important cause. Don't hesitate to get in touch with me if you are interested in helping or if you know someone who may be able to help.

The Future of Chronic Prostatitis Research

There has been a dramatic increase in scientific research on chronic prostatitis during the past 50 years. In 1970, there was just one scientific paper on chronic prostatitis. In 2020, the number of scientific papers on chronic prostatitis, which includes scientific studies and research reports, had grown to 111. During the past five years, there has been an average of 100 scientific papers per year. The total number of scientific papers on chronic prostatitis published during the past 50 years is 1,908. The US is a leader in many fields of medical research, including chronic prostatitis medical research. The US has six of the 11 most prolific medical journals publishing research on chronic prostatitis, including the Journal of Urology, the official journal of the American Urology Association. It has five of the top 10 researchers, followed by Germany with 3. The US, Canada, China, Italy, and Germany are among the top five leading countries in medical research on chronic prostatitis. **(2)** In terms of the treatments studied, The US has tended to focus more on conventional medical treatments such as prescription drugs, while other countries, in particular Italy, China, and Germany, have tended to focus more on alternative treatments such as supplements and lifestyle changes. In 2008, the National Institutes of Health launched A major federal government research

CHAPTER 11
The Future of the Chronic Prostatitis 360 Protocol

program called the MAPP Research Network to study the underlying causes of chronic prostatitis and pelvic pain. That research is ongoing and signals a major commitment to the ongoing large-scale research of chronic prostatitis and chronic pelvic pain.

This large body of research has made the Chronic Prostatitis 360 Protocol possible. It has provided scientific evidence for every part of the Prostatitis 360 Protocol and the scientific evidence that most conventional medical treatments are either not effective or not as effective as the alternative treatments in the Prostatitis 360 Protocol. While the scientific community has a long way to go, we understand the underlying causes of chronic prostatitis, and the research that has been done on treating the symptoms has made a great deal of progress. Some men can achieve a cure or come close to a cure, and many men with severe daily pain can achieve a dramatic life-changing reduction in their symptoms of 80% to 90% by following the Chronic Prostatitis 360 Protocol. I believe there is reason to be optimistic that the dramatic increase in chronic prostatitis research in the past five years will lead to a great deal of scientific progress in treating chronic prostatitis in the coming decade. I will update the Chronic Prostatitis 360 Protocol in future editions of this book to integrate the latest scientific findings on the treatment of chronic prostatitis as proven scientific treatment information becomes available. I also plan to write a Prostatitis 360 Protocol Diet cookbook and a version of the book adapted for Europe.

Appendix I
Chronic Pelvic Floor Dysfunction

The primary focus of this book is chronic prostatitis, which is a form of prostatitis directly associated with inflammation of the prostate. In Chapter 1, I discussed the fact that there is a distinctly different type of pelvic pain called Pelvic Floor Dysfunction (PFD) that is primarily associated with muscle spasms in the perineum and surrounding areas. Despite the fact that PFD and chronic prostatitis are very different conditions with different symptoms and underlying causes, there remains a great deal of confusion among urologists and patients about the two conditions, with PFD often being mislabeled as prostatitis. Given this confusion, I concluded that it was necessary to provide information about the treatment of chronic pelvic floor dysfunction. Pelvic floor dysfunction or PFD falls under the chronic pelvic pain syndrome (CPPS) part of the chronic prostatitis/chronic pelvic pain syndrome CP/CPPS name used by medical researchers. It is also sometimes simply known as pelvic floor pain. This Appendix is dedicated to treating chronic pelvic floor pain with a treatment program that is

Appendix I
Chronic Pelvic Floor Dysfunction

largely based on the Wise-Anderson protocol developed in the 1990s. The Wise-Anderson protocol is widely regarded as the most effective treatment protocol for PFD. This appendix is intended to provide an introduction to the Wise-Anderson protocol and provide additional steps you can take to enhance the proven benefits of the protocol. It is not an alternative to carefully studying and implementing the actual Wise-Anderson protocol. This appendix will address the unique and specific testing and diagnosis of PFD as well as diet, nutraceutical, and lifestyle changes that may help treat chronic pelvic floor dysfunction in addition to the Wise-Anderson Protocol.

Understanding Pelvic Floor Dysfunction

The primary symptom of chronic prostatitis is pain in the prostate and urethra caused by inflammation of the prostate. The primary symptom of pelvic floor dysfunction is pain of the pelvic floor caused by anxiety and muscle tension and spasms of pelvic floor muscles in the perineum or area between the anus and the scrotum. While there are several overlapping symptoms between these two conditions, such as ED and urination problems, the two very different primary symptoms clearly identify the two conditions as different. The lumping together of these two conditions under the name chronic prostatitis / chronic pelvic pain syndrome or CP/CPPS is unfortunate and confusing for many urologists and patients, but among scientific researchers and experts in the field, there is a clear distinction in the diagnosis, treatment, and scientific research of the two conditions.

The best and simplest way to start to determine whether you have chronic prostatitis or pelvic floor dysfunction is to complete the CPSI questionnaire. The first question is, "Have you experienced any pain or discomfort during the last week in the following areas?" A. area between the rectum and testicles. If your answer is yes, there is a strong likelihood that pelvic floor pain is the issue. This is especially true if the answer is no to the same question regarding the penis. You can also largely rule out chronic prostatitis related to the prostate. Pain is the primary symptom for 93% of men with chronic prostatitis, and almost by definition, that pain is in the penis or prostate. It is rare for men with chronic prostatitis to experience pain or any significant pain in the pelvic floor. Both conditions often include bladder issues, testicle pain, ED, and urination symptoms. What sets them apart is the location of the pain, which is the primary symptom. If you have not completed the CPSI questionnaire, if you complete it now and add up your total score, you can compare the rate of improvement from various treatments to calculate; for example, a 5-point reduction in total score would impact you based on your particular score. If your total score is 30, a 5-point reduction is not significant, whereas if your total score is 15, a 5-point reduction is a dramatic improvement in your symptoms.

Diagnosis

The diagnosis of pelvic floor dysfunction (PFD) involves the examination and testing of pain, urinary, and sexual issues, which are the primary symptoms of the condition. The diagnostic process should include the following major steps:

Physical examination of the pelvic floor
In this exam, the doctor or physical therapist feels and presses on the public floor muscles to determine if they are tight, tender, or painful to the touch. This is normally the best indicator of pelvic floor dysfunction.

Physical examination and medical history review

Appendix I
Chronic Pelvic Floor Dysfunction

After carefully reviewing the patient's medical history, the urologist should perform a thorough medical examination of the entire pelvic area, Including the perineum, scrotum, penis, and anus, and a digital rectal exam (DRE) of the prostate to identify any unusual masses, areas of tenderness, abnormalities, and areas of unusual muscle tension. The goal is to identify or rule out issues such as hernias, cysts, cancers, etc. And pinpoint areas of muscle tension and tenderness. The physical examination and medical history review should also consider and rule out the possibility of pelvic floor dysfunction, which is primarily associated with constipation and the health of the digestive tract. It should also look for pudendal nerve entrapment and pain as possible causes or contributing factors.

Pelvic ultrasound

A physical examination should be followed up with an ultrasound of the lower pelvis to identify any abnormalities that cannot be determined by a physical examination alone and analyze the masses and abnormalities found during the physical examination.

Urinalysis

A complete urine analysis and urine culture should be performed to identify and rule out any infection or inflammation-related issues.

Urination Testing

This is testing to analyze urination-related symptoms. A uroflow to measure the strength if you are in the flow. Any bladder urine retention test to determine any post-urination retention of urine in the bladder.

Erectile Dysfunction Evaluation

This should include a complete history of sexual issues, physical examination of the sex organs, testing of penal sensation, assessment of nighttime erections, and measurement of blood flow in and out of the penis. CPPS can cause ED or make a pre-existing ED worse.

Treatment Plan

Treatment for PFD has an overall high success rate with the primary symptom of pain in the pelvic floor as well as most of the secondary symptoms, such as ED and urination issues. Not all men completely resolve their symptoms, but most men dramatically reduce their symptoms.

No single treatment or monotherapy will work in most cases. PFD requires a multimodal treatment protocol that combines several different types of treatments. The Wise-Anderson Protocol is a three-part treatment program.

Part 1: Trigger Point Release

The trigger point release is a physical therapy treatment program designed to teach the patient a manual self-treatment technique for 'stretching, loosening, and lengthening the contracted tissue inside and outside the pelvic floor (1). In their book, *A Headache of the Pelvis*, Doctors Wise and Anderson provide a detailed description of trigger point release. However, they strongly recommend completing in-person or online training in trigger point release techniques. This is especially important when performing the technique inside the pelvic floor. However, the book provides detailed descriptions of trigger point release physical therapy, including diagrams. The authors report that many individuals have seen significant improvement in their symptoms by reading and implementing the treatments in the book alone.

Appendix I
Chronic Pelvic Floor Dysfunction

Physical Therapy

Most of the physical therapy treatments for PFD available around the country are based to some extent on the Wise-Anderson Protocol model and typically involve 10 sessions with a physical therapist who specializes or has significant experience with PFD physical therapy. Many of the studies done on physical therapy for pelvic floor pain are based on these 10-session treatment programs. Patients receive physical therapy and training on how to conduct an ongoing in-home physical therapy program. Most health insurance plans offered by PPOs and HMOs will pay for this session, typically a 10-week program with a referral from an in-network urologist. Some urologists have established referral relationships with physical therapists who offer treatment for chronic pelvic pain.

It is important to note that most of these ten-week programs do not include key elements of the Wise- Anderson protocol, such as relaxation techniques and biofeedback as important elements of the protocol. The protocol dedicates two hours of relaxation techniques per day initially and an hour a day thereafter. This is important because it treats the underlying cause of pelvic floor pain and tension, which is stress that is stored in the pelvic region, just as many men store pain in their neck and have chronic stress headaches. In fact, the book written by David Wise and Rodney Anderson about the Wise-Anderson treatment program for PFD is entitled "A Headache in the Pelvis." The book makes the case that the underlying cause of CPPS pain is anxiety that is "stored" or "carried" in the pelvis. (8) Biofeedback is another key protocol element that is not normally included in the typical 10-week program. Biofeedback alone as a monotherapy has been proven in several scientific studies to improve PFD symptoms significantly. A 2005 biofeedback study showed an average 51% decline in symptoms on the NIH-CPSI symptom scores for men with CPPS or

PFD. (9) Biofeedback and an intensive, professionally led long-term relaxation program must be added to the typical 10-week program to achieve the full benefits of the protocol.

Finally, the typical 10-week program is just the starting point in a long-term 6 to 12-month protocol that includes ongoing daily exercise, stretching, relaxation techniques, and the addition of biofeedback and working with a professional in stress management. The wise Anderson treatment protocol at Stanford University, for example, is either an intensive 6-month or 12-month program of weekly sessions with professionals at a treatment center in the Bay Area. This protocol is also part of a larger lifelong stress management and lifestyle change that a man with PFD must make for long-term success. This includes diet, exercise, stress management, and other lifestyle changes that we discuss later in this chapter, as well as chapters later in the book dedicated to making these changes.

These 10-week physical therapy programs, combined with carefully studying and following the detailed instructions in the Headache in the Pelvis book, are the best option if you cannot afford the on-site or in-home online Wise-Anderson training programs discussed below.

Part 2: Extended Paradoxical Relaxation

Extended Paradoxical Relaxation involves a series of relaxation techniques designed to address the chronic stress that is the underlying cause of chronic pelvic muscle tension. The book provides detailed step-by-step instructions on these relaxation techniques. Stress management programs typically require professional instruction, but you may be able to achieve significant results by carefully studying and practicing the relaxation techniques in the book.

Appendix I
Chronic Pelvic Floor Dysfunction

Part 3: Understanding How Your Attitude Affects Your Condition

Part 3 discusses a series of steps you can take to manage your attitude and your response to your chronic pelvic pain symptoms. The primary focus is on cognitive behavior therapy but also includes biofeedback, managing sexual habits, yoga, and massage, as well as managing constipation, IBS, bowel movement pain, and more. You can implement many of the components of Part 3 on your own, but some of them, such as cognitive behavior therapy and biofeedback, may require professional help. Part 3 also addresses obstacles to successfully implementing parts 1 and 2 of the protocol, such as pain catastrophizing.

Wise-Anderson Protocol Training Programs

The Wise-Anderson protocol was originally developed 20 years ago by Dr Wise, a psychologist, and Dr Anderson, a urologist at Stanford University. At first, it was available at the Stanford University campus as an on-site 6-day clinic. Today, it is available as an on-site 6-day clinic led by Dr. Wise in Santa Rosa, CA, in the Bay Area, a 60-day in-home online program, and by reading the book by Wise and Anderson, "A Headache in the pelvis." The 6-day clinic combines all-day private and group sessions for 10 to 15 students led by Dr. Wise and a physical therapist. The goal is to train each student to continue a six-month in-home program based on the training we received at the clinic. The fee for the program is $3,950 plus travel expenses for the six-day stay in Santa Rosa, CA. Health insurance may reimburse you for approximately $1000 for the physical therapy component of the clinic, depending on the type of health insurance you have and their reimbursement policy. The training program is also available as a 60-day, in-home online program with telephone hotline support. The home program includes a Kindle tablet with 104 instructional videos preloaded, an FDA-approved internal trigger point wand, and a 650-page instruction manual. The fee for the home program is $3,250. The home program is generally not covered by health insurance. Many participants in the on-site clinic and the home program recommend that you combine those programs with regular ongoing treatment by the physical therapist who follows the physical therapy program of the Wise-Anderson protocol, ideally with a physical therapist who has experience with the Wise-Anderson protocol and the use of the trigger point wand.

The best place to start is by reading the book written by Wise and Anderson, "A Headache in the pelvis." The authors report that some readers of the book have dramatically reduced their symptoms by following the instructions in the book, and some have been cured. However, the authors believe that most men need extensive training to benefit from the protocol. If you can't afford the training programs, the book may be your only option, and a good option, especially if you combine it with some physical therapy sessions based on the book.

Wise-Anderson Protocol Research

The Wise-Anderson protocol has been studied in a dozen RCT and non-RCT trials done in the past 15 years and consistently shows a 70 to 80% success rate in reducing symptoms. Typically, these studies show approximately 50% of the patients see substantial improvement, and another 20% see moderate improvement. A meta-analysis of eight studies involving 280 patients showed an overall average improvement of 8.8 points on the CPSI symptom scale. The average improvement was a 31% reduction in symptoms. Patients with severe symptoms saw an average improvement of 26%, and

Appendix I
Chronic Pelvic Floor Dysfunction

patients with moderate symptoms saw an average improvement of 40%. (1)

Acupuncture

Acupuncture is one the most widely studied and scientifically proven forms of non-drug pain treatment used by doctors who specialize in pain management. It has been used to treat the pain of chronic prostatitis and chronic PFD for over 20 years in the US and around the world. Two recent meta-analyses of 24 studies showed significant improvements in pain, quality of life, and urination on the CPSI symptoms scale. Most of these studies report a "significant" improvement in 50 to 70% of the men studied. (10) (11) A typical treatment plan consists of 10 to 12 weekly 30-minute sessions followed by monthly sessions as needed if the treatment is effective. In the US, men are typically referred to a pain management specialist by either a urologist or primary care doctor who, in turn, either has an acupuncturist on staff or works with an acupuncture provider. Health insurance companies, HMOs, and PPOs will typically approve acupuncture treatment CPPS/PFD with a referral from a pain management specialist, but in many cases, they limit the total number of treatment sessions to 8 or 10. The chapter on pain management discusses acupuncture in additional detail as part of a wide range of pain management options for both chronic prostatitis of the prostate and chronic pelvic floor dysfunction.

Prescription Medications

Several PFD prescription medications have been studied, including 5mg daily Cialis, Botox, Diazepam (Vallum), and Cyclobenzaprine. All these medications act as muscle relaxers in one form or another. Cialis has proven to be effective as a long-term treatment.

Cialis

Cialis is the most extensively studied and scientifically proven of these prescription medications. A meta-analysis of 17 studies done since 2013 concluded that 5 mg of Cialis is an effective treatment for PFD, with significant reductions in pain and urinary symptoms as well as significantly improved ED. (3) These studies show that Cialis is most effective when taken for six months or more. A 2020 15-month study found a 12.9-point reduction in overall CPSI scores, with 92% of the patients showing improvement. (2) Studies done for 12 weeks or less typically show a much lower point reduction in overall CPSI scores in the 6-point range and a response rate of approximately 50%.

Other:

Botox injections have shown improvements in pelvic floor pain for women and prostate pain in men. However, a meta-analysis of 13 RCT studies and five non-RCT studies has shown little or no benefit to pelvic floor pain in men. (4) Diazepam is used off-label for pelvic pain in women. Cyclobenzaprine (Flexeril) has been widely studied and used as a short-term treatment for pelvic pain in women. There is some but very limited experience using it for pelvic pain in men with mixed results.

Nutraceuticals for Pelvic Floor Pain

Nutraceuticals have been widely studied for prostate-related prostatitis and pelvic pain in women, but there is little scientific research about the use of supplements for chronic pelvic floor pain in men. There is limited evidence that the following supplements are beneficial for men with pelvic floor pain.

Appendix I
Chronic Pelvic Floor Dysfunction

Quercetin

There is some research on the use of Quercetin for pelvic floor pain with some evidence of symptom improvement. A 2011 study found that quercetin was effective in improving the symptoms of pelvic floor pain. (5) There have been several studies that have looked at the use of nutraceuticals, including quercetin, flower pollen, and saw palmetto, for men with both prostate and pelvic floor-related pain. But unfortunately, they do not break out the results by type of prostatitis. We can only infer that the high overall success rate means that both groups of men benefited. The most common dose used in studies is 500 milligrams, taken twice daily. The best dietary sources of quercetin are capers, red onion, and buckwheat.

Magnesium

Magnesium has been widely studied as a natural muscle relaxer. It has been used in combination formulas to treat pelvic floor pain and tension in women with some success. Relaxing the pelvic floor muscles is an important goal for any treatment protocol for pelvic floor pain. Magnesium should be taken with calcium in a 2-to-1 ratio. The typical combinations are 1000 mg calcium and 500 mg magnesium or 1,200 mg and 600 mg, respectively. The glycinate version of magnesium is better absorbed and easier in the stomach than the carbonate version. Dietary sources of magnesium include leafy greens such as spinach, figs, avocado, raspberries, nuts, and seeds.

L-Arginine

L-arginine is a natural relaxer of the pelvic floor, bladder, and urethra that has some of the same benefits as a 5 mg daily Cialis treatment and may enhance them. It is also widely used as a natural treatment for ED with pycnogenol or grape seed extract. The typical dose is 500 mg twice a day.

Omega-3
Fish oil and vitamin D are two important supplements that most men are deficient in. They play a role in managing stress and lowering pain.

The PFD Diet
Chronic inflammation is important in causing chronic pain and creating a greater sensitivity to pain. Therefore, it is believed that anti-inflammatory diets that remove inflammatory foods and increase inflammation-lowering foods can play an important role in reducing inflammation throughout the body, including the pelvic region, and lowering pain, including pelvic floor pain. (7) Chapter 3 discusses a detailed anti-inflammation diet plan. While it may not be necessary to follow the strict anti-inflammation diet in Chapter 3, many of the main components of that diet are relevant to individuals with chronic pelvic pain syndrome / pelvic floor pain

Highly inflammatory foods
The first step is to remove highly inflammatory foods from the diet. Research on chronic prostatitis and pelvic floor pain has shown that the following foods are particularly inflammatory: alcohol, caffeine, spicy and acidic foods, added sugar, carbonated drinks, artificial sweeteners, and highly processed meats such as sausages, cold cuts, and bacon. Removing alcohol is particularly important. Research done during the past 20 years has consistently shown that alcohol is the single greatest trigger of symptoms, such as pain in both chronic prostatitis and chronic pelvic pain syndrome / pelvic floor pain. For most men, that means completely abstaining from alcohol except for

Appendix I
Chronic Pelvic Floor Dysfunction

1 or 2 drinks on a few rare special occasions such as weddings, anniversaries, and holidays. It typically takes 6 to 8 weeks to see some improvement in pain, and if someone is a heavy drinker, it may take three months or more.

Foods that lower inflammation

Several categories of foods proactively lower inflammation. These anti-inflammatory foods include leafy greens; extra virgin olive oil; berries such as blueberries; cruciferous vegetables such as broccoli and cauliflower; fatty fish such as salmon, sardines, and tuna; nuts and seeds; vitamin A-rich foods such as sweet potatoes and carrots; and zinc-containing foods such as oatmeal and lentils.

High Fiber Diet

A high-fiber diet can improve digestive tract health, which plays a role in lowering inflammation throughout the body, including the pelvic area. It can play a direct role in reducing IBS, constipation, and diarrhea, which directly contribute to reducing pain and tension in the pelvic region. High-fiber foods include fresh fruits and vegetables, oatmeal, ground flax seeds, and organic psyllium husk. A good daily breakfast routine combines 4 tablespoons of oatmeal with one tablespoon each of ground flaxseed and psyllium husk cooked in hot water and topped with blueberries.

Lifestyle Changes

Lifestyle changes play an important role in the long-term success of treating CPPS. They help with the overall long-term stress, inflammation, and pain management of the condition. Lifestyle changes, along with the diet changes discussed above, dramatically reduce the symptoms of CPPS. A Three-month study done in 2014 evaluated 13 diet and lifestyle changes and their impact on CPPS symptoms. (12) These changes included:

- Diet changes: no alcohol, caffeine, or hot/spicy foods
- Increased fiber: more daily fruits and vegetables
- Avoiding a sedentary life: Aerobic exercise: walking, swimming, etc. 30 min. / day
- Limit long periods of sitting: use a donut-shaped cushion and stand up every 30 min.
- Daily hot baths
- Sexual habits: Avoid ejaculation more than twice a day, do not abstain from ejaculation for more than 4 days, and avoid *coitus interruptus*.
- Avoid sports/activities that cause perineum pressure: bike riding, rowing, horseback riding, etc.

The study showed a 63% reduction in the overall CPSI symptom score. While this is a dramatic improvement in symptoms, it's important to recognize that making these diet and lifestyle changes is difficult, especially changes such as abstaining from alcohol and caffeine. This is illustrated by the fact that 21% of the study participants dropped out of the study. It may also take more than three months for some men to see the full benefit of these diet and lifestyle changes. However, for men who have struggled with severe chronic CPPS symptoms for a long time and who don't see a significant immediate benefit from physical therapy and acupuncture, this is another important option that can play an important role in an overall treatment program to provide symptom relief. Chapter 5, which focuses on lifestyle changes, addresses implementing this lifestyle program in greater detail.

APPENDIX II
Foods and Drinks that irritate the bladder

All alcoholic drinks
Apples
Apple sauce
Cantaloupe
Carbonated beverages
Cherries
Chili's, spicy foods with cumin or ginger
Hungarian hot paprika
Chutney
Citrus fruits
Coffee (accept no acid)
Cranberries
Grapes
Lemon juice
 Papaya
Peaches

Pickles
Watermelon rind
Persimmons
Pineapple
Plums
Rhubarb
Pomegranate
Strawberries
Tea (except sun tea)
Tomatoes (except Ace VF55 or Creole)
Vinegar

Foods High in Tyrosine, Tyramine, Tryptophan, and Aspartate to be Avoided

Avocados
Bananas
Beer
Canned Figs
Champagne
Cheeses (Accept Velveeta, ricotta, mozzarella, cream cheese, String cheese, cottage cheese)
Chicken livers
Chocolate (except carbo & white)
Corned beef
Eggplant
Fava beans
Lima beans
Mayonnaise
NutraSweet
Nuts (except pine nuts)

APPENDIX II
Foods and Drinks that irritate the bladder

Onions (except shallots and green onions)
Pickled Herring
Prunes
Raisins
Rye bread
Saccharin
Sour cream
Soy sauce
Worcestershire sauce
Wines
Yogurt (except frozen)
Vitamins buffered with aspartate

Substitutes and Alternatives

1. Small amounts of cooked onions are allowed. Raw onions are not allowed. Green onions and shallots are acceptable.
2. Alcohol and wine can be used in sauces if reduced (boiled down)
3. White chocolate and carbs are good alternatives to chocolate.
4. The zest of oranges and limes can be used as a flavoring.
5. Processed cheese can be substituted for aged cheese.
6. Sun tea can be used as an alternative to regular tea. Sun tea is made by leaving tea bags in a large jar of cold water in the sun for several hours.
7. Acid-free decaffeinated coffee may be an acceptable alternative to regular coffee. Tyler's Coffee makes a 100% acid-free decaffeinated coffee. Coffee substitutes such as Kava and Rombouta are also available.

REFERENCES

CHAPTER 1

1. Nickel JC, Downey J, Hunter D, Clark J. Prevalence of prostatitis-like symptoms in a population-based study using the National Institutes of Health chronic prostatitis symptom index. J Urol. 2001 Mar;165(3):842-5.

2. Krieger JN, Lee SW, Jeon J, Cheah PY, Liong ML, Riley DE. Epidemiology of prostatitis. Int J Antimicrob Agents. 2008 Feb;31 Suppl 1(Suppl 1):S85-90. doi: 10.1016/j.ijantimicag.2007.08.028. Epub 2007 Dec 31.

3. Wallner LP, Clemens JQ, Sarma AV. Prevalence of and risk factors for prostatitis in African American men: the Flint Men's Health Study. Prostate. 2009 Jan 1;69(1):24-32. doi: 10.1002/pros.20846. PMID: 18802926; PMCID: PMC3857999.

4. Mehik A, Hellström P, Lukkarinen O, Sarpola A, Järvelin M. Epidemiology of prostatitis in Finnish men: a population-based cross-sectional study. BJU Int. 2000 Sep;86(4):443-8. doi: 10.1046/j.1464-410x.2000.00836.x. PMID: 10971269.

5. Roberts RO, Lieber MM, Rhodes T, Girman CJ, Bostwick DG, Jacobsen SJ. Prevalence of a physician-assigned

REFERENCES

diagnosis of prostatitis: the Olmsted County Study of Urinary Symptoms and Health Status Among Men. Urology. 1998 Apr;51(4):578-84. doi: 10.1016/s0090-4295(98)00034-x. PMID: 9586610.

6. Ku JH, Kim SW, Paick JS. Epidemiologic risk factors for chronic prostatitis. Int J Androl. 2005 Dec;28(6):317-27. doi: 10.1111/j.1365-2605.2005.00560.x. PMID: 16300663.

7. Null, Gary, Power Aging, Pages 94-98, New American Library Penguin Books, 2003

8. Chen Y, Li J, Hu Y, Zhang H, Yang X, Jiang Y, Yao Z, Chen Y, Gao Y, Tan A, Liao M, Lu Z, Wu C, Xian X, Wei S, Zhang Z, Chen W, Wei GH, Wang Q, Mo Z. Multi-factors including Inflammatory/Immune, Hormones, Tumor-related Proteins and Nutrition associated with Chronic Prostatitis NIH IIIa+b and IV based on FAMHES project. Sci Rep. 2017 Aug 22;7(1):9143. doi: 10.1038/s41598-017-09751-8. PMID: 28831136; PMCID: PMC5567298.

CHAPTER 2

1. Nickel JC. Perplexing problem of persistently painful prostatitis. Rev Urol. 1999 Summer;1(3):160-9. PMID: 16985790; PMCID: PMC1477525.
2. Stamatiou K, Magri V, Perletti G, Samara E, Christopoulos G, Trinchieri A. How urologists deal with chronic prostatitis. The preliminary results of a Mediterranean survey. Arch Ital Urol

Androl. 2020 Dec 21;92(4). doi: 10.4081/aiua.2020.4.353. PMID: 33348966.

3. Ornish, Dean "Dr. Dean Ornish's Program for Reversing Heart Disease" RandomHouse, 1996

4. Urology Care Foundation Website, Chronic Prostatitis Treatment, August 14, 2023

5. Research Protocol: Newer Medications for Lower Urinary Tract Symptoms (LUTS) Associated with Benign Prostatic Hyperplasia (BPH). Content last reviewed in December 2019. Effective Health Care Program, Agency for Healthcare Research and Quality, Rockville, MD. Published online: April 21, 1995

6. M. A. ALZAHRANI, S. BINSALEH1, O. SAFAR2, M. ALMURAYYI3, A. ABOUKHSHABA4 , B. O. HAKAMI5, S. ALBARMAN6, A. ALFAKHRI7 AND R. ALMANNIE, Treatment of Chronic Prostatitis with Phosphodiesterase Type 5 Inhibitors, Current Trends in Pharmaceutical and Biomedical Science, Indian J Pharm Sci 2022:84(5) Spl Issue "67-78"

7. Tawfik AM, Radwan MH, Abdulmonem M, Abo-Elenen M, Elgamal SA, Aboufarha MO. Tadalafil monotherapy in management of chronic prostatitis/chronic pelvic pain syndrome: a randomized double-blind placebo controlled clinical trial. World J Urol. 2022 Oct;40(10):2505-2511. doi: 10.1007/s00345-022-04074-4. Epub 2022 Jul 8. Erratum in: World J Urol. 2022 Oct;40(10):2513-2514. doi:

REFERENCES

10.1007/s00345-022-04128-7. PMID: 35802142; PMCID: PMC9512753.

8. Anas M, EL-Hefnawy A, Shoma A. MP15-09 TADALAFIL VERSUS COMBINED TAMSOLUSIN AND CIPROFLOXACIN FOR TREATMENT OF CHRONIC PELVIC PAIN SYNDROME: A RANDOMIZED CONTROLLED TRIAL. Journal of Urology [Internet]. 2023 Apr 1 [cited 2024 Oct 24];209(Supplement 4):e195.

9. Pineault K, Ray S, Gabrielson A, Herati AS. Phosphodiesterase type 5 inhibitor therapy provides sustained relief of symptoms among patients with chronic pelvic pain syndrome. Transl Androl Urol 2020;9(2):391-397. doi: 10.21037/tau.2020.03.05

10. Matsukawa Y, Naito Y, Funahashi Y, Ishida S, Fujita T, Tochigi K, Kato M, Gotoh M. Comparison of cernitin pollen extract vs tadalafil therapy for refractory chronic prostatitis/chronic pelvic pain syndrome: A randomized, prospective study. Neurourol Urodyn. 2020 Sep;39(7):1994-2002. doi: 10.1002/nau.24454. Epub 2020 Jul 10. PMID: 32648985.

11. Matsukawa Y, Naito Y, Funahashi Y, Ishida S, Fujita T, Tochigi K, Kato M, Gotoh M. Comparison of cernitin pollen extract vs. tadalafil therapy for refractory chronic prostatitis/chronic pelvic pain syndrome: A randomized, prospective study. Neurourol Urodyn. 2020 Sep;39(7):1994-2002. doi: 10.1002/nau.24454. Epub 2020 Jul 10. PMID: 32648985.

12. Bryk DJ, Shoskes DA. Using the UPOINT system to manage men with chronic pelvic pain syndrome. Arab J Urol. 2021 Jul 23;19(3):387-393. doi: 10.1080/2090598X.2021.1955546. PMID: 34552790; PMCID: PMC8451687.

13. Chen CH, Tyagi P, Chuang YC. Promise and the Pharmacological Mechanism of Botulinum Toxin A in Chronic Prostatitis Syndrome. Toxins (Basel). 2019 Oct 11;11(10):586. doi: 10.3390/toxins11100586. PMID: 31614473; PMCID: PMC6832516. Sandhu J, Tu HYV. Recent advances in managing chronic prostatitis/chronic pelvic pain syndrome. F1000Res. 2017 Sep 25;6:F1000 Faculty Rev-1747. doi: 10.12688/f1000research.10558.1. PMID: 29034074; PMCID: PMC5615772.

14. Falahatkar S, Shahab E, Gholamjani Moghaddam K, Kazemnezhad E. Transurethral intraprostatic injection of botulinum neurotoxin type A for the treatment of chronic prostatitis/chronic pelvic pain syndrome: results of a prospective pilot double-blind and randomized placebo-controlled study. BJU Int. 2015 Oct;116(4):641-9. doi: 10.1111/bju.12951. Epub 2015 May 25. PMID: 25307409.

15. Pan J, Jin S, Xie Q, Wang Y, Wu Z, Sun J, Guo TP, Zhang D. Acupuncture for Chronic Prostatitis or Chronic Pelvic Pain Syndrome: An Updated Systematic Review and Meta-Analysis. Pain Res Manag. 2023 Mar 14;2023:7754876. doi: 10.1155/2023/7754876. PMID: 36960418; PMCID: PMC10030225.

16. Qin Z, Guo J, Chen H, Wu J. Acupuncture for Chronic Prostatitis/Chronic Pelvic Pain Syndrome: A GRADE-assessed

REFERENCES

Systematic Review and Meta-analysis. Eur Urol Open Sci. 2022 Oct 26;46:55-67. doi: 10.1016/j.euros.2022.10.005. PMID: 36506258; PMCID: PMC9732484.

17. Sahin S, Bicer M, Eren GA, Tas S, Tugcu V, Tasci AI, Cek M. Acupuncture relieves symptoms in chronic prostatitis/chronic pelvic pain syndrome: a randomized, sham-controlled trial. Prostate Cancer Prostatic Dis. 2015 Sep;18(3):249-54. doi: 10.1038/pcan.2015.13. Epub 2015 May 5. PMID: 25939517.

18. Urology Care Foundation Website, Chronic Prostatitis Treatment, August 14, 2023

CHAPTER 3

1. Nickel JC. Alpha-blockers for the treatment of prostatitis-like syndromes. Rev Urol. 2006;8 Suppl 4(Suppl 4):S26-34. PMID: 17215998; PMCID: PMC1765040.

2. M. A. ALZAHRANI, S. BINSALEH1, O. SAFAR2, M. ALMURAYYI3, A. ABOUKHSHABA4 , B. O. HAKAMI5, S. ALBARMAN6, A. ALFAKHRI7 AND R. ALMANNIE, Treatment of Chronic Prostatitis with Phosphodiesterase Type 5 Inhibitors, Current Trends in Pharmaceutical and Biomedical Science, Indian J Pharm Sci 2022:84(5) Spl Issue "67-78"

3. Tawfik AM, Radwan MH, Abdulmonem M, Abo-Elenen M, Elgamal SA, Aboufarha MO. Tadalafil monotherapy in the management of chronic prostatitis/chronic pelvic pain syndrome: a randomized, double-blind placebo-controlled

clinical trial. World J Urol. 2022 Oct;40(10):2505-2511. doi: 10.1007/s00345-022-04074-4. Epub 2022 Jul 8. Erratum in: World J Urol. 2022 Oct;40(10):2513-2514. doi: 10.1007/s00345-022-04128-7. PMID: 35802142; PMCID: PMC9512753.

4. Anas M, EL-Hefnawy A, Shoma A. MP15-09 TADALAFIL VERSUS COMBINED TAMSOLUSIN AND CIPROFLOXACIN FOR TREATMENT OF CHRONIC PELVIC PAIN SYNDROME: A RANDOMIZED CONTROLLED TRIAL. Journal of Urology [Internet]. 2023 Apr 1 [cited 2024 Oct 24];209(Supplement 4):e195.

5. Pineault K, Ray S, Gabrielson A, Herati AS. Phosphodiesterase type 5 inhibitor therapy provides sustained relief of symptoms among patients with chronic pelvic pain syndrome. Transl Androl Urol 2020;9(2):391-397. doi: 10.21037/tau.2020.03.05

6. Matsukawa Y, Naito Y, Funahashi Y, Ishida S, Fujita T, Tochigi K, Kato M, Gotoh M. Comparison of cernitin pollen extract vs. tadalafil therapy for refractory chronic prostatitis/chronic pelvic pain syndrome: A randomized, prospective study. Neurourol Urodyn. 2020 Sep;39(7):1994-2002. doi: 10.1002/nau.24454. Epub 2020 Jul 10. PMID: 32648985.

7. Bryk DJ, Shoskes DA. Using the UPOINT system to manage men with chronic pelvic pain syndrome. Arab J Urol. 2021 Jul 23;19(3):387-393. doi: 10.1080/2090598X.2021.1955546. PMID: 34552790; PMCID: PMC8451687.

REFERENCES

8. Chen CH, Tyagi P, Chuang YC. Promise and the Pharmacological Mechanism of Botulinum Toxin A in Chronic Prostatitis Syndrome. Toxins (Basel). 2019 Oct 11;11(10):586. doi: 10.3390/toxins11100586. PMID: 31614473; PMCID: PMC6832516. Sandhu J, Tu HYV. Recent advances in managing chronic prostatitis/chronic pelvic pain syndrome. F1000Res. 2017 Sep 25;6:F1000 Faculty Rev-1747. doi: 10.12688/f1000research.10558.1. PMID: 29034074; PMCID: PMC5615772.

9. Falahatkar S, Shahab E, Gholamjani Moghaddam K, Kazemnezhad E. Transurethral intraprostatic injection of botulinum neurotoxin type A for the treatment of chronic prostatitis/chronic pelvic pain syndrome: results of a prospective pilot double-blind and randomized placebo-controlled study. BJU Int. 2015 Oct;116(4):641-9. doi: 10.1111/bju.12951. Epub 2015 May 25. PMID: 25307409.

10. Pan J, Jin S, Xie Q, Wang Y, Wu Z, Sun J, Guo TP, Zhang D. Acupuncture for Chronic Prostatitis or Chronic Pelvic Pain Syndrome: An Updated Systematic Review and Meta-Analysis. Pain Res Manag. 2023 Mar 14;2023:7754876. doi: 10.1155/2023/7754876. PMID: 36960418; PMCID: PMC10030225.

11. Qin Z, Guo J, Chen H, Wu J. Acupuncture for Chronic Prostatitis/Chronic Pelvic Pain Syndrome: A GRADE-assessed Systematic Review and Meta-analysis. Eur Urol Open Sci. 2022 Oct 26;46:55-67. doi: 10.1016/j.euros.2022.10.005. PMID: 36506258; PMCID: PMC9732484.

12. Sahin S, Bicer M, Eren GA, Tas S, Tugcu V, Tasci AI, Cek M. Acupuncture relieves symptoms in chronic prostatitis/chronic pelvic pain syndrome: a randomized, sham-controlled trial. Prostate Cancer Prostatic Dis. 2015 Sep;18(3):249-54. doi: 10.1038/pcan.2015.13. Epub 2015 May 5. PMID: 25939517.

CHAPTER 4

1. Krisiloff, Milton, "A Dietary Cure For Prostatitis and the Ureteral Syndrome" Infectious Disease in Clinical Practice: March-April 202 – Volume 11 Issue 3 – p 107 – 110.

2. Roberts RO, et al. A Review of Clinical and pathological prostatitis syndromes. Urology 1997 (6) 809=821.

3. Powell NB, Powell EB, Thomas OC, Queng JT, McGovern JP. Allergy of the Lower Urinary Tract. Journal of Urology [Internet]. 1972 Apr 1 [cited 2024 Nov 21];107(4):631–

CHAPTER 5

1. Cai T, Verze P, La Rocca R, Anceschi U, De Nunzio C, Mirone V. The role of flower pollen extract in managing patients affected by chronic prostatitis/chronic pelvic pain syndrome: a comprehensive analysis of all published clinical trials. BMC Urol. 2017 Apr 21;17(1):32. doi: 10.1186/s12894-017-0223-5. PMID: 28431537; PMCID: PMC5401347

REFERENCES

2. Buck, A.C., Rees, R.W.M., and Ebeling, L., "Treatment of Chronic Prostatitis and Prostatodynia with Pollen Extract", Br J Urol 64:496-499, 1989.

3. Elist J. Effects of pollen extract preparation Prostat/Poltit on lower urinary tract symptoms in patients with chronic nonbacterial prostatitis/chronic pelvic pain syndrome: a randomized, double-blind, placebo-controlled study. Urology. 2006 Jan;67(1):60-3. doi:

4. 10.1016/j.urology.2005.07.035. PMID: 16413333.

5. Rugendorf, F.W., Weidner, W., Eberling, L., and Buck, A.C., "Results of treatment with pollen extract (Cernilton (R Mark)) in prostatodynia and chronic prostatitis" Br J Urol, 71:433-438, 1993.

6. Cai T, Luciani LG, Caola I, Mondaini N, Malossini G, Lanzafame P, Mazzoli S, Bartoletti R. Effects of pollen extract in association with vitamins (DEPROX 500®) for pain relief in patients affected by chronic prostatitis/chronic pelvic pain syndrome: results from a pilot study. Urologia. 2013 Apr 24;80 Suppl 22:5-10. doi: 10.5301/RU.2013.10597. Epub 2013 Jan 16. PMID: 23334883.

7. Chughtai, Bilal[1]; Bhojani, Naeem[2]; Zorn, Kevin C.[2]; Elterman, Dean[3]. Variability of Commercial Saw Palmetto–Based Supplements for the Management of Benign Prostatic Hyperplasia/Lower Urinary Tract Symptoms. JU

Open Plus 1(8):e00037, August 2023. | DOI: 10.1097/JU9.0000000000000040

8. Iwamura H, Koie T, Soma O, Matsumoto T, Imai A, Hatakeyama S, Yoneyama T, Hashimoto Y, Ohyama C. Eviprostat has an identical effect compared to pollen extract (Cernilton) in patients with chronic prostatitis/chronic pelvic pain syndrome: a randomized, prospective study. BMC Urol. 2015 Dec 7;15:120. doi: 10.1186/s12894-015-0115-5. PMID: 26643109; PMCID: PMC4672535.

9. Reissigl A, Pointner J, Marberger M, et al. Multicenter Austrian trial on safety and efficacy of phytotherapy in the treatment of chronic prostatitis/chronic pelvic pain syndrome. *J Urol.* 2004;174(suppl) abstract 115

10. Zhang K, Guo RQ, Chen SW, Chen B, Xue XB, Chen S, Huang J, Liu M, Tian Y, Zuo L, Chen M, Zhou LQ. The efficacy and safety of Serenoa repens extract for the treatment of patients with chronic prostatitis/chronic pelvic pain syndrome: a multicenter, randomized, double-blind, placebo-controlled trial. World J Urol. 2021 Sep;39(9):3489-3495. doi: 10.1007/s00345-020-03577-2. Epub 2021 Jan 16. PMID: 33452912; PMCID: PMC8510895.

11. Lambertini, L.; Sandulli, A.; Salamone, V.; Bacchiani, M.; Giudici, S.; Massaro, E.; Cadenar, A.; Mariottini, R.; Coco, S.; Bardina, L.; et al. Efficacy and Safety of a Natural Supplement Containing Serenoa Repens, Solanum

REFERENCES

Lycopersicum, Lycopene, and Bromelain in Reducing Symptoms of Chronic Prostatitis/Chronic Pelvic Pain Syndrome: A Prospective Cohort Study in 250 Patients. *Uro* **2023**, *3*, 199-207.

12. Strum, Stephen B. 2021. "Serenoa Repens (Saw Palmetto) for Lower Urinary Tract Symptoms (LUTS): The Evidence for Efficacy and Safety of Lipidosterolic Extracts. Part III" *Uro* 1, no. 3: 155-179. https://doi.org/10.3390/uro1030017

13. Pavone C, Abbadessa D, Tarantino ML, et al. Associating Serenoa Repens, Urtica Dioica and Pinus Pinaster. Safety and Efficacy in the Treatment of Lower Urinary Tract Symptoms. Prospective Study on 320 Patients. *Urologia Journal*. 2010;77(1):43-51.

14. Morgia, G., Mucciardi, G., Galì, A., Madonia, M., Marchese, F., Di Benedetto, A., ... & Magno, C. (2010). Treatment of chronic prostatitis/chronic pelvic pain syndrome category IIIA with Serenoa repens plus selenium and lycopene (profluss®) versus S. repens alone: An Italian randomized multicenter-controlled study. *Urologia internationalis*, *84*(4), 400-406.

15. Macchione N, Bernardini P, Piacentini I, Mangiarotti B, Del Nero A. Flower Pollen Extract in Association with Vitamins (Deprox 500®) Versus Serenoa repens in Chronic Prostatitis/Chronic Pelvic Pain Syndrome: A Comparative Analysis of Two Different Treatments. Antiinflamm Antiallergy Agents Med Chem. 2019;18(2):151-161. doi:

10.2174/1871523018666181128164252. PMID: 30488800; PMCID: PMC6751341.

16. Kirschner-Hermanns R, Funk P, Leistner N. WS PRO 160 I 120 mg (a combination of sabal and urtica extract) in patients with LUTS related to BPH. Ther Adv Urol. 2019 Oct 11;11:1756287219879533. doi: 10.1177/1756287219879533. PMID: 31656534; PMCID: PMC6791037.

17. Shoskes DA, Zeitlin SI, Shahed A, Rajfer J. Quercetin in men with category III chronic prostatitis: a preliminary prospective, double-blind, placebo-controlled trial. Urology. 1999 Dec;54(6):960-3. doi: 10.1016/s0090-4295(99)00358-1. PMID: 10604689.

18. Shoskes DA, Nickel JC, Kattan MW. Phenotypically directed multimodal therapy for chronic prostatitis/chronic pelvic pain syndrome: a prospective study using UPOINT. Urology. 2010 Jun;75(6):1249-53. doi: 10.1016/j.urology.2010.01.021. Epub 2010 Apr 3. PMID: 20363491.

19. Curtis Nickel J, Shoskes D, Roehrborn CG, Moyad M. Nutraceuticals in Prostate Disease: The Urologist's Role. Rev Urol. 2008 Summer;10(3):192-206. PMID: 18836556; PMCID: PMC2556486.

20. Nickel JC. Alpha-blockers for the treatment of prostatitis-like syndromes. Rev Urol. 2006;8 Suppl 4(Suppl 4):S26-34. PMID: 17215998; PMCID: PMC1765040.

REFERENCES

21. Safarinejad MR. Urtica dioica for treatment of benign prostatic hyperplasia: a prospective, randomized, double-blind, placebo-controlled, crossover study. J Herb Pharmacother. 2005;5(4):1-11. PMID: 16635963.

22. Kirschner-Hermanns R, Funk P, Leistner N. WS PRO 160 I 120 mg (a combination of sabal and urtica extract) in patients with LUTS related to BPH. Ther Adv Urol. 2019 Oct 11;11:1756287219879533. doi: 10.1177/1756287219879533. PMID: 31656534; PMCID: PMC6791037.

23. Oelke M, Berges R, Schläfke S, Burkart M. Fixed-dose combination PRO 160/120 of sabal and urtica extracts improves nocturia in men with LUTS suggestive of BPH: re-evaluation of four controlled clinical studies. World J Urol. 2014 Oct;32(5):1149-54. doi: 10.1007/s00345-014-1338-x. Epub 2014 Jun 18. PMID: 24938176.

24. Lopatkin N, Sivkov A, Schläfke S, Funk P, Medvedev A, Engelmann U. Efficacy and safety of a combination of Sabal and Urtica extract in lower urinary tract symptoms-- long-term follow-up of a placebo-controlled, double-blind, multicenter trial. Int Urol Nephrol. 2007;39(4):1137-46. doi: 10.1007/s11255-006-9173-7. Epub 2007 Feb 15. PMID: 18038253.

25. Friederich M, Theurer C, Schiebel-Schlosser G. Prosta Fink Forte -kapseln in der behandlung der benignen prostatahyperplasie. Eine multizentrische Anwendungsbeobachtung an 2245 patienten] [Prosta Fink

Forte capsules in the treatment of benign prostatic hyperplasia. Multicentric surveillance study in 2245 patients]. Forsch Komplementarmed Klass Naturheilkd. 2000 Aug;7(4):200-4. German. doi: 10.1159/000021344. PMID: 11025395.

26. Nishimura M, Ohkawara T, Sato H, Takeda H, Nishihira J. Pumpkin Seed Oil Extracted From Cucurbita maxima Improves Urinary Disorder in Human Overactive Bladder. J Tradit Complement Med. 2014 Jan;4(1):72-4. doi: 10.4103/2225-4110.124355. PMID: 24872936; PMCID: PMC4032845.

27. Bongseok Shim, Hyewon Jeong, Sara Lee, Sehee Hwang, Byeongseok Moon, Charlotte Storni, A randomized double-blind placebo-controlled clinical trial of a product containing pumpkin seed extract and soy germ extract to improve overactive bladder-related voiding dysfunction and quality of life, Journal of Functional Foods, Volume 8, 2014, pages 111-117, ISSN 1756-4646.

28. Martin Leibbrand, Simone Siefer, Christiane Schön, Tania Perrinjaquet-Moccetti, Albert Kompek, Anca Csernich, Franz Bucar, and Matthias Heinrich Kreuter Effects of an Oil-Free Hydroethanolic Pumpkin Seed Extract on Symptom Frequency and Severity in Men with Benign Prostatic Hyperplasia: A Pilot Study in Humans, Journal of Medicinal Food 2019 22:6, 551-559

29. Damiano R, Cai T, Fornara P, Franzese CA, Leonardi R, Mirone V. The role of Cucurbita pepo in the management

REFERENCES

of patients affected by lower urinary tract symptoms due to benign prostatic hyperplasia: A narrative review. Arch Ital Urol Androl. 2016 Jul 4;88(2):136-43. doi: 10.4081/aiua.2016.2.136. PMID: 27377091.

30. Gomez Y et al. Zinc levels in prostatic fluid of patients with prostate pathologies. *Invest Clin* 2007 Sep; 48(3): 287-94

31. Bao B, Prasad AS, Beck FW, Fitzgerald JT, Snell D, Bao GW, Singh T, Cardozo LJ. Zinc decreases C-reactive protein, lipid peroxidation, and inflammatory cytokines in elderly subjects: a potential implication of zinc as an atheroprotective agent. Am J Clin Nutr. 2010 Jun;91(6):1634-41. doi: 10.3945/ajcn.2009.28836. Epub 2010 Apr 28. PMID: 20427734; PMCID: PMC2869512.

32. Lombardo, F., Effects of a dietary supplement on chronic pelvic pain syndrome (Category IIIA), leucocytospermia and semen parameters, 07 November 2011https://doi.org/10.1111/j.1439-0272.2011.01248.x

33. Hui-Juan C, Shi-Bing L, Jian-Ping L, Bin W, Hai-Song L, Ji-Sheng W, Si-Qi G, Yu-Tian Z, Heng-Heng D, Chun-Yu Z. Qian lie an suppository (prostant) for chronic prostatitis: A systematic review and meta-analysis of randomized controlled trials. Medicine (Baltimore). 2019 Apr;98(14): e15072. doi: 10.1097/MD.0000000000015072. PMID: 30946356; PMCID: PMC6456157.

34. Gorpynchenko, I. et al. The Clinical and Immunologic Effects of Acetylcysteine in the Treatment of Chronic

Abacterial Prostatitis. Journal of Allergy and Clinical Immunology, AB30 Volume 145, Issue 2, Supplement AB30 February 2020

CHAPTER 6

1. Gallo L. Effectiveness of diet, sexual habits and lifestyle modifications on treatment of chronic pelvic pain syndrome. Prostate Cancer Prostatic Dis. 2014 Sep;17(3):238-45. doi: 10.1038/pcan.2014.18. Epub 2014 May 13. PMID: 24819236.

2. Giubilei G, Mondaini N, Minervini A, Saieva C, Lapini A, Serni S, Bartoletti R, Carini M. Physical activity of men with chronic prostatitis/chronic pelvic pain syndrome not satisfied with conventional treatments--could it represent a valid option? The physical activity and male pelvic pain trial: a double-blind, randomized study. J Urol. 2007 Jan;177(1):159-65. doi: 10.1016/j.juro.2006.08.107. PMID: 17162029.

3. Zhang R, Chomistek AK, Dimitrakoff JD, Giovannucci EL, Willett WC, Rosner BA, Wu K. Physical activity and chronic prostatitis/chronic pelvic pain syndrome. Med Sci Sports Exerc. 2015 Apr;47(4):757-64. doi: 10.1249/MSS.0000000000000472. PMID: 25116086; PMCID: PMC4324388.

4. Cramer H, Lauche R, Anheyer D, Pilkington K, de Manincor M, Dobos G, Ward L. Yoga for anxiety: A

REFERENCES

systematic review and meta-analysis of randomized controlled trials. Depress Anxiety. 2018 Sep;35(9):830-843. doi: 10.1002/da.22762. Epub 2018 Apr 26. PMID: 29697885.

5. Mark S. Nestor, MS, Lawson, A., Fischer, D; Improving the mental health and well-being of health care providers using the transcendental meditation technique during the COVID-19 pandemic: a parallel population study PLOS One., March 3, 2023, https://doi.org/10.1371/journal.pone.0265046

6. Goyal M, Singh S, Sibinga EM, Gould NF, Rowland-Seymour A, Sharma R, Berger Z, Sleicher D, Maron DD, Shihab HM, Ranasinghe PD, Linn S, Saha S, Bass EB, Haythornthwaite JA. Meditation programs for psychological stress and well-being: a systematic review and meta-analysis. JAMA Intern Med. 2014 Mar;174(3):357-68. doi: 10.1001/jamainternmed.2013.13018. PMID: 24395196; PMCID: PMC4142584.

7. Cui YH, Zheng Y. A meta-analysis on the efficacy and safety of St John's wort extract in depression therapy in comparison with selective serotonin reuptake inhibitors in adults. Neuropsychiatr Dis Treat. 2016 Jul 11;12:1715-23. doi: 10.2147/NDT.S106752. PMID: 27468236; PMCID: PMC4946846.

8. Shelton RC, Sloan Manning J, Barrentine LW, Tipa EV. Assessing Effects of l-Methylfolate in Depression Management: Results of a Real-World Patient Experience

Trial. Prim Care Companion CNS Disord. 2013;15(4):PCC.13m01520. doi: 10.4088/PCC.13m01520. Epub 2013 Aug 29. PMID: 24392264; PMCID: PMC3869616.

9. Cuomo A, Beccarini Crescenzi B, Bolognesi S, Goracci A, Koukouna D, Rossi R, Fagiolini A. S-Adenosylmethionine (SAMe) in major depressive disorder (MDD): a clinician-oriented systematic review. Ann Gen Psychiatry. 2020 Sep 5;19:50. doi: 10.1186/s12991-020-00298-z. PMID: 32939220; PMCID: PMC7487540.

10. Hausenblas HA, Saha D, Dubyak PJ, Anton SD. Saffron (Crocus sativus L.) and major depressive disorder: a meta-analysis of randomized clinical trials. J Integr Med. 2013 Nov;11(6):377-83. doi: 10.3736/jintegrmed2013056. PMID: 24299602; PMCID: PMC4643654.

11. St-Onge MP, Mikic A, Pietrolungo CE. Effects of Diet on Sleep Quality. Adv Nutr. 2016 Sep 15;7(5):938-49. doi: 10.3945/an.116.012336. PMID: 27633109; PMCID: PMC5015038.

12. Gallo L. Effectiveness of diet, sexual habits and lifestyle modifications on treatment of chronic pelvic pain syndrome. Prostate Cancer Prostatic Dis. 2014 Sep;17(3):238-45. doi: 10.1038/pcan.2014.18. Epub 2014 May 13. PMID: 24819236.

13. Giubilei G, Mondaini N, Minervini A, Saieva C, Lapini A, Serni S, Bartoletti R, Carini M. Physical activity of men with chronic prostatitis/chronic pelvic pain syndrome not

REFERENCES

satisfied with conventional treatments--could it represent a valid option? The physical activity and male pelvic pain trial: a double-blind, randomized study. J Urol. 2007 Jan;177(1):159-65. doi: 10.1016/j.juro.2006.08.107. PMID: 17162029.

14. Zhang R, Chomistek AK, Dimitrakoff JD, Giovannucci EL, Willett WC, Rosner BA, Wu K. Physical activity and chronic prostatitis/chronic pelvic pain syndrome. Med Sci Sports Exerc. 2015 Apr;47(4):757-64. doi: 10.1249/MSS.0000000000000472. PMID: 25116086; PMCID: PMC4324388.

15. Cramer H, Lauche R, Anheyer D, Pilkington K, de Manincor M, Dobos G, Ward L. Yoga for anxiety: A systematic review and meta-analysis of randomized controlled trials. Depress Anxiety. 2018 Sep;35(9):830-843. doi: 10.1002/da.22762. Epub 2018 Apr 26. PMID: 29697885.

16. Mark S. Nestor, MS, Lawson, A, Fischer, D; Improving the mental health and well-being of health care providers using the transcendental meditation technique during the COVID-19 pandemic: a parallel population study PLOS One., March 3, 2023, https://doi.org/10.1371/journal.pone.0265046

17. Goyal M, Singh S, Sibinga EM, Gould NF, Rowland-Seymour A, Sharma R, Berger Z, Sleicher D, Maron DD, Shihab HM, Ranasinghe PD, Linn S, Saha S, Bass EB, Haythornthwaite JA. Meditation programs for psychological stress and well-being: a systematic review

and meta-analysis. JAMA Intern Med. 2014 Mar;174(3):357-68. doi: 10.1001/jamainternmed.2013.13018. PMID: 24395196; PMCID: PMC4142584.

18. Cui YH, Zheng Y. A meta-analysis on the efficacy and safety of St John's wort extract in depression therapy in comparison with selective serotonin reuptake inhibitors in adults. Neuropsychiatr Dis Treat. 2016 Jul 11;12:1715-23. doi: 10.2147/NDT.S106752. PMID: 27468236; PMCID: PMC4946846.

19. Shelton RC, Sloan Manning J, Barrentine LW, Tipa EV. Assessing Effects of l-Methylfolate in Depression Management: Results of a Real-World Patient Experience Trial. Prim Care Companion CNS Disord. 2013;15(4):PCC.13m01520. doi: 10.4088/PCC.13m01520. Epub 2013 Aug 29. PMID: 24392264; PMCID: PMC3869616.

20. Cuomo A, Beccarini Crescenzi B, Bolognesi S, Goracci A, Koukouna D, Rossi R, Fagiolini A. *S*-Adenosylmethionine (SAMe) in major depressive disorder (MDD): a clinician-oriented systematic review. Ann Gen Psychiatry. 2020 Sep 5;19:50. doi: 10.1186/s12991-020-00298-z. PMID: 32939220; PMCID: PMC7487540.

21. Hausenblas HA, Saha D, Dubyak PJ, Anton SD. Saffron (Crocus sativus L.) and major depressive disorder: a meta-analysis of randomized clinical trials. J Integr Med. 2013 Nov;11(6):377-83. doi: 10.3736/jintegrmed2013056. PMID: 24299602; PMCID: PMC4643654.

REFERENCES

22. St-Onge MP, Mikic A, Pietrolungo CE. Effects of Diet on Sleep Quality. Adv Nutr. 2016 Sep 15;7(5):938-49. doi: 10.3945/an.116.012336. PMID: 27633109; PMCID: PMC5015038.

CHAPTER 7

35. Lang-Illievich K, Klivinyi C, Lasser C, Brenna CTA, Szilagyi IS, Bornemann-Cimenti H. Palmitoylethanolamide in the Treatment of Chronic Pain: A Systematic Review and Meta-Analysis of Double-Blind Randomized Controlled Trials. Nutrients. 2023 Mar 10;15(6):1350. doi: 10.3390/nu15061350. PMID: 36986081; PMCID: PMC10053226.

36. Stochino Loi E, Pontis A, Cofelice V, Pirarba S, Fais MF, Daniilidis A, Melis I, Paoletti AM, Angioni S. Effect of ultra micronized-palmitoylethanolamide and co-micronized palmitoylethanolamide/polydatin on chronic pelvic pain and quality of life in endometriosis patients: An open-label pilot study. Int J Womens Health. 2019 Aug 12;11:443-449. doi: 10.2147/IJWH.S204275. PMID: 31496832; PMCID: PMC6697671.

37. Indraccolo, U., et al., Micronized palmitoylethanolamide/ *trans*-polydatin treatment of endometriosis-related pain: a meta-analysis, Ann Ist Super Sanità 2017 | Vol. 53, No. 2: 125-134 DOI: 10.4415/ANN_17_02_08

38. Gubbiotti, M., Novel Formulation of Palmitoylethanolamide/ Serenoa Repens in the treatment of Chronic Prostatitis/ Chronic Pelvic Pain Syndrome, Scientific Open Discussion Session 21 2019 Abstract 338.

39. Lin, K.Y.-H.; Chang, Y.-C.; Lu, W.-C.; Kotha, P.; Chen, Y.-H.; Tu, C.-H. Analgesic Efficacy of Acupuncture on Chronic Pelvic Pain: A Systemic Review and Meta-Analysis Study. *Healthcare* **2023**, *11*,830. https://doi.org/10.3390/ healthcare11060830, Academic Editor: Edward J. Pavlik, Published: 11 March 2023

40. Sun, Y., et al., Efficacy of Acupuncture for Chronic Prostatitis/Pelvic Pain Syndrome, Annuals of Internal Medicine, October 2021

41. Chen CH, Tyagi P, Chuang YC. Promise and the Pharmacological Mechanism of Botulinum Toxin A in Chronic Prostatitis Syndrome. Toxins (Basel). 2019 Oct 11;11(10):586. doi: 10.3390/toxins11100586. PMID: 31614473; PMCID: PMC6832516. Sandhu J, Tu HYV. Recent advances in managing chronic

42. Sahin S, Bicer M, Eren GA, Tas S, Tugcu V, Tasci AI, Cek M. Acupuncture relieves symptoms in chronic prostatitis/chronic pelvic pain syndrome: a randomized, sham-controlled trial. Prostate Cancer Prostatic Dis. 2015 Sep;18(3):249-54. doi: 10.1038/pcan.2015.13. Epub 2015 May 5. PMID: 25939517.

43. Chen CH, Tyagi P, Chuang YC. Promise and the Pharmacological Mechanism of Botulinum Toxin A in

REFERENCES

>Chronic Prostatitis Syndrome. Toxins (Basel). 2019 Oct 11;11(10):586. doi: 10.3390/toxins11100586. PMID: 31614473; PMCID: PMC6832516. Sandhu J, Tu HYV. Recent advances in managing chronic prostatitis/chronic pelvic pain syndrome. F1000Res. 2017 Sep 25;6:F1000 Faculty Rev-1747. doi: 10.12688/f1000research.10558.1. PMID: 29034074; PMCID: PMC5615772.

44. Qin, Z., et al. Oral pharmacological treatments for chronic prostatitis/chronic pelvic pain syndrome: A systematic prostatitis/chronic pelvic pain syndrome: A systematic review and network meta-analysis of randomized controlled trials. eClinical Medicine 2022;48: 101457 Published online 20 May 2022

45. Zhang M, Li H, Ji Z, Dong D, Yan S. Clinical study of duloxetine hydrochloride combined with doxazosin for the treatment of pain disorder in chronic prostatitis/chronic pelvic pain syndrome: An observational study. Medicine (Baltimore). 2017 Mar;96(10):e6243. doi: 10.1097/MD.0000000000006243. PMID: 28272220; PMCID: PMC5348168.

46. De Rose et al., THE ROLE OF MEPARTRICIN IN CATEGORY III CHRONIC NONBACTERIAL PROSTATITIS/ CHRONIC PELVIC PAIN SYNDROME (CPPS): A RANDOMIZED PROSPECTIVE PLACEBO-CONTROLLED TRIAL, The Journal of Urology, Vol. 183, Is. 45, April 2010.

47. Agarwal, M., et al., "Gabapentenoids in pain management in urological chronic pelvic pain syndrome: Gabapentin or pregabalin?" AMIS 10 February 2017

48. Christos Papandreou, Petros Skapinakis, Dimitrios Giannakis, Nikolaos Sofikitis, Venetsanos Mavreas, "Antidepressant Drugs for Chronic Urological Pelvic Pain: An Evidence-Based Review", *Advances in Urology*, vol. 2009, Article ID 797031, 9 pages, 2009.

49. Dimitrkove, J., et al., MEMANTINE IN THE ALLEVIATION OF SYMPTOMS OF CHRONIC PELVIC PAIN SYNDROME: A RANDOMIZED, DOUBLE-BLIND PLACEBO-CONTROLLED TRIAL, The Journal of Urology Vol. 181, April 26, 2009.

CHAPTER 8

1. Miller JM, Garcia CE, Hortsch SB, Guo Y, Schimpf MO. Does Instruction to Eliminate Coffee, Tea, Alcohol, Carbonated, and Artificially Sweetened Beverages Improve Lower Urinary Tract Symptoms?: A Prospective Trial. J Wound Ostomy Continence Nurs. 2016 Jan-Feb;43(1):69-79. doi: 10.1097/WON.0000000000000197. PMID: 26727685; PMCID: PMC4799659.

2. Safarinejad MR. Urtica dioica for treatment of benign prostatic hyperplasia: a prospective, randomized, double-blind, placebo-controlled, crossover study. J Herb Pharmacother. 2005;5(4):1-11. PMID: 16635963.

REFERENCES

3. Kirschner-Hermanns R, Funk P, Leistner N. WS PRO 160 I 120 mg (a combination of sabal and urtica extract) in patients with LUTS related to BPH. Ther Adv Urol. 2019 Oct 11;11:1756287219879533. doi: 10.1177/1756287219879533. PMID: 31656534; PMCID: PMC6791037.

4. Oelke M, Berges R, Schläfke S, Burkart M. Fixed-dose combination PRO 160/120 of sabal and urtica extracts improves nocturia in men with LUTS suggestive of BPH: re-evaluation of four controlled clinical studies. World J Urol. 2014 Oct;32(5):1149-54. doi: 10.1007/s00345-014-1338-x. Epub 2014 Jun 18. PMID: 24938176.

5. Friederich M, Theurer C, Schiebel-Schlosser G. Prosta Fink Forte -kapseln in der behandlung der benignen prostatahyperplasie. Eine multizentrische Anwendungsbeobachtung an 2245 patienten] [Prosta Fink Forte capsules in the treatment of benign prostatic hyperplasia. Multicentric surveillance study in 2245 patients]. Forsch Komplementarmed Klass Naturheilkd. 2000 Aug;7(4):200-4. German. doi: 10.1159/000021344. PMID: 11025395.

6. Nishimura M, Ohkawara T, Sato H, Takeda H, Nishihira J. Pumpkin Seed Oil Extracted From Cucurbita maxima Improves Urinary Disorder in Human Overactive Bladder. J Tradit Complement Med. 2014 Jan;4(1):72-4. doi: 10.4103/2225-4110.124355. PMID: 24872936; PMCID: PMC4032845.

7. Bongseok Shim, Hyewon Jeong, Sara Lee, Sehee Hwang, Byeongseok Moon, Charlotte Storni, A randomized double-

blind placebo-controlled clinical trial of a product containing pumpkin seed extract and soy germ extract to improve overactive bladder-related voiding dysfunction and quality of life, Journal of Functional Foods, Volume 8, 2014, pages 111-117, ISSN 1756-4646.

8. Martin Leibbrand, Simone Siefer, Christiane Schön, Tania Perrinjaquet-Moccetti, Albert Kompek, Anca Csernich, Franz Bucar, and Matthias Heinrich Kreuter <u>Effects of an Oil-Free Hydroethanolic Pumpkin Seed Extract on Symptom Frequency and Severity in Men with Benign Prostatic Hyperplasia: A Pilot Study in Humans</u>, Journal of Medicinal Food 2019 22:6, 551-559

9. Damiano R, Cai T, Fornara P, Franzese CA, Leonardi R, Mirone V. The role of Cucurbita pepo in the management of patients affected by lower urinary tract symptoms due to benign prostatic hyperplasia: A narrative review. Arch Ital Urol Androl. 2016 Jul 4;88(2):136-43. doi: 10.4081/aiua.2016.2.136. PMID: 27377091.

10. Damiano R, Cai T, Fornara P, Franzese CA, Leonardi R, Mirone V. The role of Cucurbita pepo in the management of patients affected by lower urinary tract symptoms due to benign prostatic hyperplasia: A narrative review. Arch Ital Urol Androl. 2016 Jul 4;88(2):136-43. doi: 10.4081/aiua.2016.2.136. PMID: 27377091.

11. Cicero, A.F.G.; Allkanjari, O.; Busetto, G.M.; Cai, T.; Largana, G.; Magri, V.; Perletti, G.; Della Cuna, F.S.R.; Russo, G.I.;

REFERENCES

12. Kutwin,P.;Falkowski,P.;Lowicki,R.;Borowiecka-Kutwin,M.;Konecki,T. Are we sentenced to pharmacotherapy? Promising role of lycopene and vitamin

13. A in benign urologic conditions. *Nutrients* **2022**, *14*, 859.

14. Carrasco, C.; Blanco, L.; Abengozar, A.; Beatriz-Rodiguez, A. Effects of lycopene-enriched, organic, extra virgin olive oil on benign prostatic hyperplasia: A pilot study. *Altern. Ther. Health Med.* **2022**, *28*, 8–15.

15. Wilt T, Ishani A, Mac Donald R, Rutks I, Stark G. Pygeum africanum for benign prostatic hyperplasia. Cochrane Database Syst Rev. 2002;1998(1): CD001044. doi: 10.1002/14651858.CD001044. PMID: 11869585; PMCID: PMC7032619.

CHAPTER 9

1. Hongjun, L., et al., Prevalence of sexual dysfunction in men with chronic prostatitis/chronic pelvic pain syndrome: a meta-analysis., World Journal of Urology 34(7) July 2016. DOI:10.1007/s00345-015-1720-3

2. Shiri R, Koskimäki J, Hakama M, Häkkinen J, Tammela TL, Huhtala H, Auvinen A. Prevalence and severity of erectile dysfunction in 50 to 75-year-old Finnish men. J Urol. 2003 Dec;170(6 Pt 1):2342-4. doi:

3. 10.1097/01.ju.0000090963.88752.84. PMID: 14634411.

4. Mitka, M. et al, Some men who take Viagra die – Why? <u>JAMA The Journal of the American Medical Association</u> March 2000 283(5):590, 593

5. Cohen JS. Comparison of FDA reports of patient deaths associated with sildenafil and with injectable alprostadil. Ann Pharmacother. 2001 Mar;35(3):285-8. doi: 10.1345/aph.10218. PMID: 11261524.

6. Maiorino MI, Bellastella G, Esposito K. Lifestyle modifications and erectile dysfunction: what can be expected? Asian J Androl. 2015 Jan-Feb;17(1):5-10. doi: 10.4103/1008-682X.137687. PMID: 25248655; PMCID: PMC4291878.

7. Biddinger, K., et al. Association of Habitual Alcohol Intake with Risk of Cardiovascular Disease March 25, 2022, doi:10.1001/jamanetworkopen.2022.3849

8. Liu Q, Zhang Y, Wang J, Li S, Cheng Y, Guo J, Tang Y, Zeng H, Zhu Z. Erectile Dysfunction and Depression: A Systematic Review and Meta-Analysis. J Sex Med. 2018 Aug;15(8):1073-1082. doi: 10.1016/j.jsxm.2018.05.016. Epub 2018 Jun 28. PMID: 29960891.

9. Schmidt, H.M., Munder, T., Gerger, H., Frühauf, S. and Barth, J. (2014), PDE-5 Inhibitors and Psychological Intervention. J Sex Med, 11: 1376-1391.

10. Kalaitzidou I, Venetikou MS, Konstadinidis K, Artemiadis AK, Chrousos G, Darviri C. Stress management and erectile dysfunction: a pilot comparative study. Andrologia.

REFERENCES

2014 Aug;46(6):698-702. doi: 10.1111/and.12129. Epub 2013 Jul 3. PMID: 23822751.

11. Gerbild H, Larsen CM, Graugaard C, Areskoug Josefsson K. Physical Activity to Improve Erectile Function: A Systematic Review of Intervention Studies. Sex Med. 2018 Jun;6(2):75-89. doi: 10.1016/j.esxm.2018.02.001. Epub 2018 Apr 13. PMID: 29661646; PMCID: PMC5960035.

12. Hicks, C., et al., Association of Peripheral Neuropathy with Erectile Dysfunction in US
Am J Med. 2021 February; 134(2): 282–284. doi:10.1016/j.amjmed.2020.07.015.

13. Sansone A, Cignarelli A, Sansone M, Romanelli F, Corona G, Gianfrilli D, Isidori A, Giorgino F, Lenzi A. Serum Homocysteine Levels in Men with and without Erectile Dysfunction: A Systematic Review and Meta-Analysis. Int J Endocrinol. 2018 Aug 7;2018:7424792. doi: 10.1155/2018/7424792. PMID: 30158975; PMCID: PMC6109500.

14. Bauer SR, Breyer BN, Stampfer MJ, Rimm EB, Giovannucci EL, Kenfield SA. Association of Diet With Erectile Dysfunction Among Men in the Health Professionals Follow-up Study. JAMA Netw Open. 2020 Nov 2;3(11):e2021701. doi: 10.1001/jamanetworkopen.2020.21701. PMID: 33185675; PMCID: PMC7666422.

15. Angelis A, Chrysohoou C, Tzorovili E, Laina A, Xydis P, Terzis I, Ioakeimidis N, Aznaouridis K, Vlachopoulos C,

Tsioufis K. The Mediterranean Diet Benefits on Cardiovascular Hemodynamics and Erectile Function in Chronic Heart Failure, Male Patients by Decoding Central and Peripheral Vessel Rheology. Nutrients. 2020 Dec 30;13(1):108. doi: 10.3390/nu13010108. PMID: 33396861; PMCID: PMC7824543.

16. Di Francesco S, Tenaglia RL. Mediterranean diet and erectile dysfunction: a current perspective. Cent European J Urol. 2017 Jun 30;70(2):185-187. doi: 10.5173/ceju.2017.1356. Epub 2017 Jun 11. PMID: 28721287; PMCID: PMC5510347.

17. Petre, Gabriel Cosmin, Francesco Francini-Pesenti, Amerigo Vitagliano, Giuseppe Grande, Alberto Ferlin, and Andrea Garolla. 2023. "Dietary Supplements for Erectile Dysfunction: Analysis of Marketed Products, Systematic Review, Meta-Analysis and Rational Use" *Nutrients* 15, no. 17: 3677. https://doi.org/10.3390/nu15173677

18. Rhim HC, Kim MS, Park YJ, Choi WS, Park HK, Kim HG, Kim A, Paick SH. The Potential Role of Arginine Supplements on Erectile Dysfunction: A Systemic Review and Meta-Analysis. J Sex Med. 2019 Feb;16(2):223-234. doi: 10.1016/j.jsxm.2018.12.002. Erratum in: J Sex Med. 2020 Mar;17(3):560. PMID: 30770070.

19. Menafra D, de Angelis C, Garifalos F, Mazzella M, Galdiero G, Piscopo M, Castoro M, Verde N, Pivonello C, Simeoli C, Auriemma RS, Colao A, Pivonello R. Long-term high-dose L-arginine supplementation in patients with vasculogenic erectile dysfunction: a multicentre, double-

REFERENCES

blind, randomized, placebo-controlled clinical trial. J Endocrinol Invest. 2022 May;45(5):941-961. doi:10.1007/s40618-021-01704-3. Epub 2022 Jan 1. PMID: 34973154; PMCID: PMC8995264.

20. Barassi, A. et al., Levels of L-arginine and L-citrulline in patients with erectile dysfunction of different etiology Andrology 12-Sept-2106, doi: 10.1111/andr.12293

21. Tian, Y., efficacy of El arginine and Pycnogenol® in the treatment of male erectile dysfunction: a systematic review and met up analysis, Front. Endocrinol. Volume 14 – 2023 | doi: 10.3389 /fendo.2023.1211720

22. Stanislavov R, Nikolova V. Treatment of erectile dysfunction with pycnogenol and L-arginine. J Sex Marital Ther. 2003 May-Jun;29(3):207-13. doi: 10.1080/00926230390155104. PMID: 12851125.

23. Stanislavov R, Rohdewald P. Improvement of erectile function by a combination of French maritime pine bark and roburins with amino acids. Minerva Urol Nefrol. 2015 Mar;67(1):27-32. PMID: 25664962.

24. Wibisono, D., et al, Efficacy of tadalafil and l-arginine combination therapy compared with tadalafil-only for the treatment of erectile dysfunction: A systematic review and meta-analysis Bali Medical Journal (*Bali MedJ*) 2023, Volume 12, Number 1: 312-318 P-ISSN.2089-1180, E-ISSN: 2302-2914

25. Gallo L, Pecoraro S, Sarnacchiaro P, Silvani M, Antonini G. The Daily Therapy With L-Arginine 2,500 mg and Tadalafil 5 mg in Combination and Monotherapy for the Treatment of Erectile Dysfunction: A Prospective, Randomized Multicentre Study. Sex Med. 2020 Jun;8(2):178-185. doi: 10.1016/j.esxm.2020.02.003. Epub 2020 Mar 16. PMID: 32192966; PMCID: PMC7261690.

26. Abu El-Hamd M, Hegazy EM. Comparison of the clinical efficacy of daily use of L-arginine, tadalafil, and combined L-arginine with tadalafil in the treatment of elderly patients with erectile dysfunction. Andrologia. 2020 Aug;52(7):e13640. doi: 10.1111/and.13640. Epub 2020 May 22. PMID: 32441833.

27. Frajese GV, Pozzi F, Frajese G. Tadalafil in the treatment of erectile dysfunction; an overview of the clinical evidence. Clin Interv Aging. 2006;1(4):439-49. doi: 10.2147/ciia.2006.1.4.439. PMID: 18046921; PMCID: PMC2699638.

28. Lee HW, Lee MS, Kim TH, Alraek T, Zaslawski C, Kim JW, Moon DG. Ginseng for Erectile Dysfunction: A Cochrane Systematic Review. World J Mens Health. 2022 Apr;40(2):264-269. doi: 10.5534/wjmh.210071. Epub 2021 Jun 15. PMID: 34169686; PMCID

CHAPTER 10

1. Huang X, Qin Z, Cui H, Chen J, Liu T, Zhu Y, Yuan S. Psychological factors and pain catastrophizing in men with

REFERENCES

chronic prostatitis/chronic pelvic pain syndrome (CP/CPPS): a meta-analysis. Transl Androl Urol 2020;9(2):485-493. doi: 10.21037/tau.2020.01.25

2. Kwon JK, Chang IH. Pain, catastrophizing, and depression in chronic prostatitis/chronic pelvic pain syndrome. Int Neurourol J. 2013 Jun;17(2):48-58. doi: 10.5213/inj.2013.17.2.48. Epub 2013 Jun 30. PMID: 23869268; PMCID: PMC3713242.

3. Nickel JC, Mullins C, Tripp DA. Development of an evidence-based cognitive behavioral treatment program for men with chronic prostatitis/chronic pelvic pain syndrome. World J Urol. 2008 Apr;26(2):167-72. doi: 10.1007/s00345-008-0235-6. Epub 2008 Feb 22. PMID: 18293000.

4. Kwon JK, Chang IH. Pain, catastrophizing, and depression in chronic prostatitis/chronic pelvic pain syndrome. Int Neurourol J. 2013 Jun;17(2):48-58. doi: 10.5213/inj.2013.17.2.48. Epub 2013 Jun 30. PMID: 23869268; PMCID: PMC3713242.

5. Li, Arthur Sone-Wai, Van Niekerk, Leesa, Wong, Aquina Lim Yim, Matthewson, Mandy and Garry, Michael. "Psychological management of patients with chronic prostatitis/chronic pelvic pain syndrome (CP/CPPS): a systematic review," *Scandinavian Journal of Pain*, vol. 23, no. 1, 2023, pp. 25-39.

6. Tripp DA, Nickel JC, Katz L. A feasibility trial of a cognitive-behavioral symptom management program for

chronic pelvic pain for men with refractory chronic prostatitis/chronic pelvic pain syndrome. Can Urol Assoc J. 2011 Oct;5(5):328-32. doi: 10.5489/cuaj.10201. PMID: 22031613; PMCID: PMC3202005.

7. Lackner JM, Clemens JQ, Radziwon C, Danforth TL, Ablove TS, Krasner SS, et al. Cognitive Behavioral Therapy for Chronic Pelvic Pain: What Is It and Does It Work? Journal of Urology [Internet]. 2024 Apr 1 [cited 2024 Nov 6];211(4):539–50. Available from:

8. Lee RA, West RM, Wilson JD. The response to sertraline in men with chronic pelvic pain syndrome. Sex Transm Infect. 2005 Apr;81(2):147-9. doi: 10.1136/sti.2004.010868. PMID: 15800093; PMCID: PMC1764675.

9. Zhang M, Li H, Ji Z, Dong D, Yan S. Clinical study of duloxetine hydrochloride combined with doxazosin for the treatment of pain disorder in chronic prostatitis/chronic pelvic pain syndrome: An observational study. Medicine (Baltimore). 2017 Mar;96(10):e6243. doi: 10.1097/MD.0000000000006243. PMID: 28272220; PMCID: PMC5348168.

10. Xia D, Wang P, Chen J, Wang S, Jiang H. Fluoxetine ameliorates symptoms of refractory chronic prostatitis/chronic pelvic pain syndrome. Chin Med J (Engl). 2011 Jul;124(14):2158-61. PMID: 21933619.

11. Nickel JC, Downey J, Hunter D, Clark J. Prevalence of prostatitis-like symptoms in a population-based study using

REFERENCES

the National Institutes of Health chronic prostatitis symptom index. J Urol. 2001 Mar;165(3):842-5.

12. Goyal M, Singh S, Sibinga EM, Gould NF, Rowland-Seymour A, Sharma R, Berger Z, Sleicher D, Maron DD, Shihab HM, Ranasinghe PD, Linn S, Saha S, Bass EB, Haythornthwaite JA. Meditation programs for psychological stress and well-being: a systematic review and meta-analysis. JAMA Intern Med. 2014 Mar;174(3):357-68. doi: 10.1001/jamainternmed.2013.13018. PMID: 24395196; PMCID: PMC4142584.

13. Singh B, Olds T, Curtis R, Dumuid D, Virgara R, Watson A, Szeto K, O'Connor E, Ferguson T, Eglitis E, Miatke A, Simpson CE, Maher C. Effectiveness of physical activity interventions for improving depression, anxiety, and distress: an overview of systematic reviews. Br J Sports Med. 2023 Sep;57(18):1203-1209. doi: 10.1136/bjsports-2022-106195. Epub 2023 Feb 16. PMID: 36796860; PMCID: PMC10579187.

14. Buric, I, et al., Individual differences in meditation interventions: A meta-analytic study British Journal of Health Psychology, February 2022.

15. Orme-Johnson DW, Barnes VA. Effects of the transcendental meditation technique on trait anxiety: a meta-analysis of randomized controlled trials. J Altern Complement Med. 2014 May;20(5):330-41. doi: 10.1089/acm.2013.0204. Epub 2013 Oct 9. PMID: 24107199.

16. Cramer H, Lauche R, Langhorst J, Dobos G. Yoga for depression: a systematic review and meta-analysis. Depress Anxiety. 2013 Nov;30(11):1068-83. doi: 10.1002/da.22166. Epub 2013 Aug 6. PMID: 23922209.

17. Saeed SA, Antonacci DJ, Bloch RM. Exercise, yoga, and meditation for depressive and anxiety disorders. Am Fam Physician. 2010 Apr 15;81(8):981-6. PMID: 20387774.

18. Simon NM, Hofmann SG, Rosenfield D, Hoeppner SS, Hoge EA, Bui E, Khalsa SBS. Efficacy of Yoga vs Cognitive Behavioral Therapy vs Stress Education for the Treatment of Generalized Anxiety Disorder: A Randomized Clinical Trial. JAMA Psychiatry. 2021 Jan 1;78(1):13-20. doi: 10.1001/jamapsychiatry.2020.2496. PMID: 32805013; PMCID: PMC7788465.

19. Hou WH, Chiang PT, Hsu TY, Chiu SY, Yen YC. Treatment effects of massage therapy in depressed people: a meta-analysis. J Clin Psychiatry. 2010 Jul;71(7):894-901. doi: 10.4088/JCP.09r05009blu. Epub 2010 Mar 23. PMID: 20361919.

20. Poland RE, Gertsik L, Favreau JT, Smith SI, Mirocha JM, Rao U, Daar ES. Open-label, randomized, parallel-group controlled clinical trial of massage for treatment of depression. J Altern Complement Med. 2013 Apr;19(4):334-40. doi: 10.1089/acm.2012.0058. Epub 2012 Oct 25. PMID: 23098696; PMCID: PMC3627430.

REFERENCES

21. Rapaport MH, Schettler PJ, Larson ER, Carroll D, Sharenko M, Nettles J, Kinkead B. Massage Therapy for Psychiatric Disorders. Focus (Am Psychiatr Publ). 2018 Jan;16(1):24-31. doi: 10.1176/appi.focus.20170043. Epub 2018 Jan 24. PMID: 31975897; PMCID: PMC6519566.

22. Zhao, Y. et al. The brain structure, immunometabolic, and genetic mechanisms underlying the association between lifestyle and depression. *Nat. Ment. Health* (2023).

23. Aguilar-Latorre A, Oliván-Blázquez B, Algorta GP, Serrano-Ripoll MJ, Olszewski LE, Turón-Lanuza A. One-year follow-up of the effectiveness of a lifestyle modification program as an adjuvant treatment of depression in primary care: A randomized clinical trial. J Affect Disord. 2023 Jul 1;332:231-237. doi: 10.1016/j.jad.2023.04.007. Epub 2023 Apr 11. PMID: 37054898.

24. Xiaowen Wang, Ahmed Arafa, Keyang Liu, Ehab S. Eshak, Yonghua Hu, Jia-Yi Dong, Combined healthy lifestyle and depressive symptoms: a meta-analysis of observational studies, Journal of Affective Disorders, Volume 289, 292, Pages 144-150, ISSN 0165-0327

25. Merkouris E, Mavroudi T, Miliotas D, Tsiptsios D, Serdari A, Christidi F, Doskas TK, Mueller C, Tsamakis K. Probiotics' Effects in the Treatment of Anxiety and Depression: A Comprehensive Review of 2014-2023 Clinical Trials. Microorganisms. 2024 Feb 19;12(2):411.

doi: 10.3390/microorganisms12020411. PMID: 38399815; PMCID: PMC10893170.

26. Zhang Q, Chen B, Zhang J, Dong J, Ma J, Zhang Y, Jin K, Lu J. Effect of prebiotics, probiotics, synbiotics on depression: results from a meta-analysis. BMC Psychiatry. 2023 Jun 29;23(1):477. doi: 10.1186/s12888-023-04963-x. PMID: 37386630; PMCID: PMC10308754.

27. Nikolova VL, Cleare AJ, Young AH, Stone JM. Acceptability, Tolerability, and Estimates of Putative Treatment Effects of Probiotics as Adjunctive Treatment in Patients With Depression: A Randomized Clinical Trial. JAMA Psychiatry. 2023 Aug 1;80(8):842-847. doi: 10.1001/jamapsychiatry.2023.1817. PMID: 37314797; PMCID: PMC10267847.

28. Miyaoka T, Kanayama M, Wake R, Hashioka S, Hayashida M, Nagahama M, Okazaki S, Yamashita S, Miura S, Miki H, Matsuda H, Koike M, Izuhara M, Araki T, Tsuchie K, Azis IA, Arauchi R, Abdullah RA, Oh-Nishi A, Horiguchi J. Clostridium butyricum MIYAIRI 588 as Adjunctive Therapy for Treatment-Resistant Major Depressive Disorder: A Prospective Open-Label Trial. Clin Neuropharmacol. 2018 Sep/Oct;41(5):151-155. doi: 10.1097/WNF.0000000000000299. PMID: 30234616.

29. da Silva LEM, de Santana MLP, Costa PRF, Pereira EM, Nepomuceno CMM, Queiroz VAO, de Oliveira LPM, Machado MEPDC, de Sena EP. Zinc supplementation combined with antidepressant drugs for the treatment of patients with depression: a systematic review and meta-

REFERENCES

analysis. Nutr Rev. 2021 Jan 1;79(1):1-12. doi: 10.1093/nutrit/nuaa039. PMID: 32885249.

30. Ranjbar E, Shams J, Sabetkasaei M, M-Shirazi M, Rashidkhani B, Mostafavi A, Bornak E, Nasrollahzadeh J. Effects of zinc supplementation on the efficacy of antidepressant therapy, inflammatory cytokines, and brain-derived neurotrophic factor in patients with major depression. Nutr Neurosci. 2014 Feb;17(2):65-71. doi: 10.1179/1476830513Y.0000000066. Epub 2013 Nov 26. PMID: 23602205.
31. Mehdi S, Manohar K, Shariff A, Kinattingal N, Wani SUD, Alshehri S, Imam MT, Shakeel F, Krishna KL. Omega-3 Fatty Acids Supplementation in the Treatment of Depression: An Observational Study. J Pers Med. 2023 Jan 27;13(2):224. doi: 10.3390/jpm13020224. PMID: 36836458; PMCID: PMC9962071.
32. Gao S, Khalid A, Amini-Salehi E, Radkhah N, Jamilian P, Badpeyma M, Zarezadeh M. Folate supplementation as a beneficial add-on treatment in relieving depressive symptoms: A meta-analysis of meta-analyses. Food Sci Nutr. 2024 Mar 8;12(6):3806-3818. doi: 10.1002/fsn3.4073. PMID: 38873435; PMCID: PMC11167194.

33. Almeida OP, Ford AH, Flicker L. Systematic review and meta-analysis of randomized placebo-controlled trials of folate and vitamin B12 for depression. Int Psychogeriatr. 2015 May;27(5):727-37. doi: 10.1017/S1041610215000046. Epub 2015 Feb 3. PMID: 25644193.

34. Canenguez Benitez JS, Hernandez TE, Sundararajan R, Sarwar S, Arriaga AJ, Khan AT, Matayoshi A, Quintanilla HA, Kochhar H, Alam M, Mago A, Hans A, Benitez GA. Advantages and Disadvantages of Using St. John's Wort as a Treatment for Depression. Cureus. 2022 Sep 22;14(9):e29468. doi: 10.7759/cureus.29468. PMID: 36299970; PMCID: PMC958790

35. Shelton RC, Sloan Manning J, Barrentine LW, Tipa EV. Assessing Effects of l-Methylfolate in Depression Management: Results of a Real-World Patient Experience Trial. Prim Care Companion CNS Disord. 2013;15(4):PCC.13m01520. doi: 10.4088/PCC.13m01520. Epub 2013 Aug 29. PMID: 24392264; PMCID: PMC3869616.

36. Cuomo A, Beccarini Crescenzi B, Bolognesi S, Goracci A, Koukouna D, Rossi R, Fagiolini A. *S*-Adenosylmethionine (SAMe) in major depressive disorder (MDD): a clinician-oriented systematic review. Ann Gen Psychiatry. 2020 Sep 5;19:50. doi: 10.1186/s12991-020-00298-z. PMID: 32939220; PMCID: PMC7487540.

37. Tóth B, Hegyi P, Lantos T, Szakács Z, Kerémi B, Varga G, Tenk J, Pétervári E, Balaskó M, Rumbus Z, Rakonczay Z, Bálint ER, Kiss T, Csupor D. The Efficacy of Saffron in the Treatment of Mild to Moderate Depression: A Meta-analysis. Planta Med. 2019 Jan;85(1):24-31. doi: 10.1055/a-0660-9565. Epub 2018 Jul 23. PMID: 30036891.

REFERENCES

CHAPTER 11

1. This estimate is based on a study showing that 16% of men have prostatitis and uses the total male population above age 25. There was no adjustment for the study showing that 40% of men do not seek medical help to treat their prostatitis symptoms, which implies that the percentage of men with prostatitis could be significantly higher. If so, 5 million may be a conservative estimate.

2. Liu SJ, Gao QH, Deng YJ, Zen Y, Zhao M, Guo J. Knowledge domain and emerging trends in chronic prostatitis/chronic pelvic pain syndrome from 1970 to 2020: a scientometric analysis based on VOSviewer and CiteSpace. Ann Palliat Med. 2022 May;11(5):1714-1724. doi: 10.21037/apm-21-3068. Epub 2022 Feb 9. PMID: 35144392.

About the Author

Philip Potasiak is a senior executive with an MBA from the University of Chicago and 12 years of CEO experience. In the summer of 2018, he began suffering from severe chronic prostatitis pain. After several years of enduring severe pain and trying a wide range of conventional medical treatments, including drugs and surgery, without finding relief, he decided to conduct his own research and experiment with alternative treatments.

As a result of extensive research, he discovered a solution for his chronic prostatitis based on scientifically proven natural treatments. This led to the development of the Chronic Prostatitis 360 Protocol and inspired him to write this book to help other men struggling with chronic prostatitis.

Index

A

- Abstinence, 171
- Action, 261
- Acupuncture, 74, 91, 190 — *See also: Alternative treatments*
- Acute Bacterial, 30 — *See: Bacterial*
- Adrenergic, 87 — *See: Inhibitors*
- Aerobic, 171 — *See: Exercise*
- Aerobic exercise, 262 — *See also: Exercise*
- Age, 27
- Alcohol, 108 — *See also: Alcoholic drinks*
- Alcoholic drinks, 108
- Alpha, 86 — *See: Inhibitors*
- Alternative, 73 — *See also: Complimentary Alternative Medicine*
- Alternative treatments, 9, 66 — *See also: Multimodal therapy*
- Alternatives, 82
- American diet, 16 — *See: Diet*
- American healthcare system, 20 — *See: Healthcare*
- Amitriptyline, 199 — *See also: Antidepressants*
- Antibiotics, 86, 113 — *See: Antimicrobial*
- Anticholinergic, 87 — *See: Inhibitors*
- Anti-inflammation, 104 — *See also: Inflammation*
- Antimicrobial, 67 — *See also: Antibiotics*
- Asparagus, 124 — *See: Diet*
- Asymptomatic Inflammatory Prostatitis, 31 — *See: Inflammation*

B

- Bacterial, 86 — *See also: Acute Bacterial*
- Benign prostatic hyperplasia (BPH), 4, 32, 65, 71, 105
- Bipolar disorder, 178 — *See: Mental disorders*

- Bladder, 119 — *See also: Bladder symptoms, Urination*
- Bladder symptoms, 210
- Bladder urine retention, 42, 209 — *See: Urination*
- Blood Tests, 46 — *See: Diagnosis*
- Botox, 84 — *See: Botox Prostate Injections*
- Botox Prostate Injections, 192
- BPNO, 49

C

- Caffeine, 109
- Cannabis, 190 — *See: Alternative treatments*
- Cardiovascular diseases, 227
- Case, 81 — *See: Case Study*
- Case Study, 78
- Catastrophizing, 254
- Cauliflower, 124, 125 — *See: Diet*
- Cernilton flower pollen, 90 — *See: Alternative treatments*
- Charles Darwin, 111 — *See: Evolution*
- Chronic Pelvic Floor Dysfunction, 24 — *See also: Chronic pelvic pain syndrome*
- Chronic pelvic pain syndrome (CPPS), 23, 24, 69, 82, 298
- Chronic poor sleep, 184 — *See: Insomnia*
- Chronic prostatitis, 6, 69, 82, 188 — *See also: Chronic Prostatitis Symptom Index*
- Chronic Prostatitis 360 Protocol, 3, 4, 8, 64
- Chronic Prostatitis Symptom Index (CPSI), 69, 91
- Cialis, 88, 308 — *See: Erectile dysfunction*
- Circumstances, 84
- Citrus Fruits, 113 — *See: Diet*
- Clinical depression, 270 — *See: Depression*
- Cognitive Behavior Therapy (CBT), 256
- Coitus interruptus, 171 — *See: Ejaculation*
- Committed Urologist, 67 — *See: Medical professionals*
- Communication, 260
- Complementary treatment(s), 264, 271

Index

- — *See also: Alternative treatments*
- Complimentary Alternative Medicine, 252 — *See also: Complementary treatment(s)*
- Connoisseur, 110
- Conventional medicine/treatments, 2, 3, 77, 84, 187 — *See also: Multimodal therapy*
- Cookbook, 123, 297 — *See: Diet*
- Cramping, 210 — *See: Bladder symptoms*
- C-reactive, 46 — *See: C-reactive protein*
- C-reactive protein, 106
- Cruciferous, 120 — *See: Diet*
- Cucurbita Maxima, 215
- Cucurbita Pepo, 215
- Cystoscopy, 70 — *See: Diagnosis*
- Cytokines, 177 — *See: Inflammation*

D

- Depression, 84, 177, 253 — *See also: Clinical depression*
- DHEA, 251
- Diagnosis, 40 — *See also: Blood Tests, Cystoscopy*
- Diarrhea, 106
- Dizziness, 198
- Doctors, 5, 74 — *See: Medical professionals*
- Doxazosin, 198
- Dr Daniel Shoskes, 66
- Dr Nichel, 66 — *See: Dr Nickel*
- Dr Nickel, 68
- Dr. J. Curtis Nichols, 10
- Dr. Milton Krisiloff, 103
- Dr. Ornish, 76
- Duloxetine, 198 — *See also: Antidepressants*
- Dysuria, 229 — *See: Urination*

E

- ED Superfoods, 237 — *See: Erectile dysfunction*
- Ejaculation, 37, 171 — *See also: Coitus interruptus*
- Enlarged Prostate, 211 — *See also: Benign prostatic hyperplasia*
- Erectile dysfunction (ED), 4, 84, 196, 222 — *See also: Cialis, ED Superfoods*

- Evaluation, 68 — *See: Diagnosis*
- EWST, 97
- Experience, 69
- Extended Paradoxical Relaxation, 304 — *See: Relaxation*

F

- Fiber, 121 — *See: Diet*
- Fibrinogen, 106
- Flaxseed, 122, 125 — *See: Diet*
- Framework, 15
- Frequent urination, 183 — *See: Urination*

G

- Gabapentin, 199
- Gastrointestinal, 107, 114
- General Guidelines, 123 — *See: Diet*
- Gluten, 116 — *See also: Diet, Inflammation*

H

- Headache, 198
- Health plans, 78 — *See: American healthcare system*
- Healthcare, 79 — *See: American healthcare system*
- Hemorrhoids, 106
- High blood pressure, 249 — *See: Cardiovascular diseases*
- Histamine, 116 — *See: Inflammation*
- HMO, 70, 100 — *See: Health plans*
- Holy basil, 109 — *See: Alternative treatments*
- Homocysteine, 106
- Horseradish, 109 — *See: Diet*

I

- Important treatment, 8 — *See: Multimodal therapy*
- Improve urination symptoms, 214 — *See: Urination*
- Improved Sleep, 182 — *See: Sleep, Insomnia*
- Improvement, 87
- Incontinence, 209 — *See: Bladder symptoms*
- Inflammation, 13, 33, 86, 102, 204 — *See also: Anti-inflammation, Cytokines*
- Inflammatory, 13 — *See: Inflammation*
- Inhibitors, 87 — *See also: Adrenergic, Alpha, Anticholinergic*

Index

- Injections, 95 — *See also: Botox Prostate Injections*
- Insomnia, 184 — *See: Sleep*
- Interstitial cystitis (IC), 38, 105, 203 — *See: Chronic pelvic pain syndrome*
- Interventionalist, 67 — *See: Medical professionals*

K

- Kidney failure, 249 — *See also: Cardiovascular diseases*
- Korean Ginseng, 247 — *See: Alternative treatments*

L

- Lactose intolerance, 115 — *See: Diet*
- Lifestyle changes, 110, 203, 268 — *See also: Diet, Stress management*
- Limitations, 75
- L-methyl folate, 282
- Lumped, 32
- Lycopene, 216 — *See: Diet*

M

- Major Risk Factors, 229 — *See: Risk factors*
- Management of Stress, 260 — *See also: Meditation, Relaxation*
- Massage therapy, 267 — *See also: Complementary treatment*
- MAST Cell Activation Syndrome (MCAS), 117 — *See also: Inflammation*
- Matsukawa, 90
- Medical professionals/specialists, 11, 83 — *See also: Doctors, Urologist*
- Meditation, 175, 259, 264 — *See also: Relaxation, Stress*
- Mediterranean diet, 122, 234 — *See: Diet*
- Melatonin supplement, 6 — *See: Sleep*
- Mental disorders, 249 — *See also: Depression, Bipolar disorder*
- Mepartricin, 198
- Meta-analysis tracker, 95
- Mild stress, 280 — *See: Stress*

- Multimodal therapy, 74, 104 — *See also: Important treatment, Complementary treatment*
- Muscle relaxation, 184 — *See: Relaxation*

N
- Naproxen, 106
- Natural remedies, 76 — *See: Alternative treatments*
- Neuritis, 107
- Nitric oxide, 110
- Nocturia, 208 — *See: Urination*
- Numbness, 198
- Nutritional guidelines, 122 — *See: Diet*

O
- Obesity, 249 — *See: Risk factors*
- Omega-3, 122, 125 — *See: Diet*
- Orchitis, 107
- Ovarian cancer, 249 — *See: Risk factors*
- Overactive bladder, 187, 208 — *See: Bladder symptoms*
- Oxidative stress, 112 — *See: Inflammation*

P
- Pain management, 11, 64, 115, 138 — *See also: Chronic prostatitis*
- Panic attacks, 177
- Parkinson's disease, 249
- Pelvic pain, 248 — *See: Chronic pelvic pain syndrome*
- Pelvic floor dysfunction, 24 — *See: Chronic pelvic floor dysfunction*
- Perineal pain, 31
- Physical therapy, 69, 90
- Pollen extract, 90 — *See: Alternative treatments*
- Prostatitis, 30, 84, 95 — *See: Chronic prostatitis, Acute prostatitis*
- Prostate, 171 — *See also: Benign prostatic hyperplasia*
- Prostate cancer, 248
- Prostate health, 4, 30 — *See: Benign prostatic hyperplasia*
- Prostatectomy, 32
- Prostate-specific antigen (PSA), 49 — *See: Diagnosis*
- Psychological support, 270 — *See: Mental disorders*
- Pyuria, 107

Q

- Quercetin, 124 — *See: Diet*

R

- Radiotherapy, 249
- Relaxation techniques, 259, 267 — *See also: Meditation, Stress management*
- Risk factors, 106, 229 — *See also: Obesity*
- Root causes, 79 — *See: Alternative treatments*
- Routine check-ups, 46 — *See: Healthcare*
- Rupture, 111

S

- Sedative medications, 198
- Self-care, 79 — *See: Lifestyle changes*
- Sexual dysfunction, 171, 196 — *See: Erectile dysfunction*
- Sleep, 3, 182 — *See also: Insomnia*
- Stress, 3, 260 — *See also: Stress management*
- Stress management, 4, 260, 268 — *See also: Meditation, Relaxation*
- Supplements, 117 — *See: Diet*
- Surgery, 105, 210 — *See: Prostatectomy*
- Symptom relief, 208 — *See: Chronic prostatitis*

T

- Testosterone therapy, 196
- Tadalafil, 88 — *See: Erectile dysfunction*
- Tinctures, 104 — *See: Alternative treatments*
- Therapy, 249 — *See also: Cognitive Behavior Therapy*
- Tofu, 121 — *See: Diet*

U

- Ureter, 119
- Urinary frequency, 183 — *See: Urination*
- Urinary incontinence, 209 — *See: Bladder symptoms*
- Urination, 43, 209 — *See also: Bladder symptoms, Frequent urination*
- Urinary tract infections (UTIs), 107, 119 — *See: Bladder symptoms*
- Urologist, 70, 84 — *See also: Medical professionals*

V

- Vasectomy, 11, 170

- Vitamin D, 106
- Vitamin E, 106
- Vitamin K, 116

W
- Weight loss, 124, 249 — *See: Obesity*
- Withdrawal symptoms, 198
- Work-life balance, 268 — *See: Lifestyle changes*

X
- Xerostomia, 107

Y
- Yeast infections, 107

Z
- Zinc, 122, 125 — *See: Diet*

www.ingramcontent.com/pod-product-compliance
Lightning Source LLC
Chambersburg PA
CBHW020453030426
42337CB00011B/96